The Minor Illness Manual

Fifth Edition

The Minor Illness Manual

Fifth Edition

Gina Johnson MSc MB BS MRCGP
General Practitioner

Ian Hill-Smith BSc MB BS MRCP FRCGP MD
General Practitioner

Chirag Bakhai BSc MB BS MRCGP DRCOG DGM MBA
General Practitioner

Foreword by Ravi Sharma

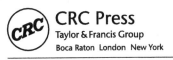

CRC Press
Taylor & Francis Group
Boca Raton London New York

CRC Press is an imprint of the
Taylor & Francis Group, an **informa** business

CRC Press
Taylor & Francis Group
6000 Broken Sound Parkway NW, Suite 300
Boca Raton, FL 33487-2742

International Standard Book Number-13: 978-1-138-49758-0 (Paperback)

Visit the Taylor & Francis Web site at
http://www.taylorandfrancis.com

and the CRC Press Web site at
http://www.crcpress.com

Contents

Contents

Foreword to the fifth edition

As the National Health Service (NHS) enters its 70th year, the concept of 'minor illness' and its treatment has changed considerably. In 2016 approximately 57 million consultations in primary care were associated with 'minor illness'; this number is predicted to rise in the future. It is widely recognised that NHS transformation is essential to meet the current needs of the public and make appropriate care readily available for patients at the earliest point of contact with a healthcare professional. The ensuing political and policy changes have provided new and exciting opportunities for all healthcare professionals to deliver care differently. This shift towards an integrated, multi-disciplinary healthcare workforce working collaboratively can only lead to improvements in the quality of patient care and a reduction in pressure on the NHS, with patients being seen by the most appropriate clinical professional in a convenient and timely manner.

Over the last decade, the role of the pharmacist has expanded radically. The drive towards new ways of working has seen pharmacists working in general practice, care homes and urgent and emergency services, enhancing the clinical services already provided by hospital and community pharmacists. As healthcare professionals extend the scope of their practice, so too does the demand to increase their level of knowledge and skills. Continuing professional development is therefore critical to delivering the best care to patients and the public, and there is a great need to have excellent resources to enable us to keep up to date.

The updated edition of *The Minor Illness Manual* therefore arrives at the perfect time to provide support for clinicians in both new and existing roles. Access to the most reliable sources of information helps support best practice, enabling pharmacists and other healthcare professionals to maintain and enhance the high quality of care we strive to provide our patients.

I congratulate the authors on their fantastic work, which will ensure all clinicians who manage the conditions covered in this book have accessible, up-to-date and evidence-based guidelines to support their work in primary care.

Ravi Sharma, M Pharm, MSc
Senior GP Practice Pharmacist and Programme Clinical Lead (Clinical Pharmacy)
– Primary Care Workforce and Infrastructure Team at NHS England

Preface to the fifth edition

In the 20 years since the first edition of this book was published, the NHS has gone through enormous changes. Now a patient with a minor illness may now be assessed in a range of different settings by a variety of healthcare professionals, including nurses, pharmacists and paramedics.

In order to distinguish major from minor illness and to manage minor illness safely, you face the challenge of learning new skills in assessment, prescribing and referral. The practical advice given in this book is designed to guide you through the diagnostic process and help you form an appropriate management plan. The text has been completely revised for this new edition, which now includes explanations of the likely major diagnoses behind the 'red flags' and the appropriate courses of action.

Please visit our website www.minorillness.co.uk, home of the National Minor Illness Centre (NMIC), for free downloads and information about our face-to-face courses and e-learning updates. You can use the voucher in the front of this book to obtain six months' free access to our members' service, which includes targeted e-mail alerts for any important changes in guidance.

Gina Johnson
Ian Hill-Smith
Chirag Bakhai

About the authors

National Minor Illness Centre (NMIC)

All of the authors have previously worked together in Kingfisher Practice, an NHS general practice near Luton Airport. In 1996, the practice designed an innovative educational programme for nurses on the management of minor illness, and in 2007, the National Minor Illness Centre (NMIC) was developed as an educational component to the practice. NMIC has received commissions from Health Education England and the Centre for Postgraduate Pharmacy Education to provide bespoke training. Over 2000 healthcare professionals (nurses, pharmacists, health visitors and paramedics) have attended NMIC courses and the NMIC Diploma is accredited by the Royal College of Nursing.

The first *Minor Illness Manual* appeared in 1997, when the notion of a non-doctor led service in general practice appeared radical. Now in its 5th edition, it has sold more than 25,000 copies: testimony to the growth, acceptance (by patients and medical staff) and success of higher-level healthcare professionals in the delivery of healthcare in a rapidly changing NHS.

Dr Gina Johnson graduated from Guy's Hospital in London in 1979 and worked as a general practitioner in Luton from 1983 to 2017. She has always been actively involved in primary care audit and research, and has published articles on a wide range of topics. She is very aware of the limitations of Western medicine, which led her to study for an MSc in medical anthropology in 2002. She is a medical acupuncturist and has an interest in holistic care.

Dr Ian Hill-Smith started publishing research papers while studying for his first degree in anatomy, before graduating in medicine from University College London, in 1980. He is both a member of the Royal College of Physicians and a fellow of the Royal College of General Practitioners. He is fascinated by fundamental science and how it can be applied to medical practice, particularly how medicines can be prescribed to best effect, which was the subject of his research MD. His previous local and national roles have led to the development of a primary care prescribing formulary, reduced medicines wastage and courses on medicines optimisation. Currently he is a member of the advisory committee on managing common infections of the National Institute for Health and Care Excellence (NICE).

Dr Chirag Bakhai discovered his enthusiasm for teaching while studying medicine at University College London, where he tutored fellow students in subjects ranging from pharmacology to statistics. Although he still makes time for one-to-one education, he also presents at conferences and events around the country. As well as working as a general practitioner, Chirag is a Clinical Director at Luton Clinical Commissioning Group and a Clinical Advisor for NHS England. He employs his evidence-based approach in improving healthcare services and is committed to empowering people to self-manage their health conditions. His teaching experience is extremely helpful in identifying and addressing learning needs across the health system and reducing unwarranted variation in standards of care.

Acknowledgements

We would like to thank the staff at the Kingfisher Practice for their support. We would also like to thank our own highly skilled minor illness nurses, both past and present (especially the pioneer, Rhona Rollings). We are grateful to the many nurses, pharmacists and paramedics who have attended our courses and seminars, who have taught us so much.

We acknowledge the excellent work of the Clinical Knowledge Summaries team in gathering together the evidence for the management of a wide range of conditions, and would like to thank them for their patience in responding to our queries and comments.

We also thank our patients for allowing us to learn from their experiences of minor illness.

CHAPTER 1

The NHS of the future: resilient, adaptive and united

Since its launch 70 years ago in 1948, the National Health Service (NHS) has been continually adapting and evolving. Some might say that these changes seem cyclical, evidenced by its seemingly perpetual reorganisation and restructuring, or the advent, removal, reintroduction and then partial abolishment of prescription charges. However, other changes seem more obviously revolutionary and necessary for its survival. The world is changing rapidly with the pace ever increasing; people's expectations, disease patterns, lifestyles, medicines and technology are very different now to when *The Minor Illness Manual's* first edition was written in 1997.

The last 20 years have seen great advances in technology, new treatments and an evolution in our approach to healthcare. Minor illness management has changed considerably. We aim to look at the whole person rather than just the disease process; we share decision-making rather than instructing; we actively seek to empower people in self-management. Meanwhile, expectations for 24/7 responsive services for non-urgent care, increasing antimicrobial resistance and sheer unprecedented demand drive the need for further change.

The issues undermining the sustainability of our health system extend globally. The pressures of a growing older population with multiple complex comorbidities, compounded by more expensive new treatments and limited resources, face the vast majority of countries previously referred to as 'more economically developed'. Other countries are very likely to follow in the coming years as their birth rates continue reducing and life expectancies further improve.

Despite these pressures, its reliance on public taxation for funding and remaining free at point-of-care, the NHS does remarkably well. Pleasingly for us working within it (and arguably because of us all), in 2017, the NHS was ranked the top healthcare system out of 11 countries analysed by the Commonwealth Fund, an international and influential healthcare think tank. Compared against North American, Australasian and European healthcare systems, the United Kingdom was judged as best overall as well as highest for equity and care processes, including prevention, safety, coordination and engagement, despite having the fourth lowest funding in terms of percentage of gross domestic product (GDP).

Our system has already recognised that, in the face of growing demand, limited resources and workforce pressures, it cannot maintain such performance without making key changes to who delivers care, how it is given and how it is organised. These changes address some of the greatest challenges facing the NHS: from the oft-publicised lack of doctors and nurses available to provide care, to the lesser known difficulties arising from outmoded internal payment structures. In this chapter, we will look at these changes to the healthcare landscape and pay particular attention to the practical considerations for minor illness management.

WHO DELIVERS CARE

Back in 1997, when the first edition of *The Minor Illness Manual* was published, minor illness was the almost-exclusive domain of the General Practitioner (GP). The work of the co-authors in teaching minor illness management to nurses was revolutionary and unorthodox. Since then, minor illness management by nurses has become commonplace. Such changes in the roles, responsibilities and composition of the primary care team are likely to continue and indeed further accelerate, with increasing diversity in skill-mix and professions represented.

The audience of *The Minor Illness Manual* is itself illustrative of the changes afoot in who delivers care. From a readership comprised of doctors and nurses a few years ago, with few exceptions, the audience has since expanded to include clinical pharmacists, paramedics and physician associates, mirroring the changes in primary care. In this section, we will examine the drivers for this expanding skill mix and its implications.

Three useful starting points are workforce recruitment, primary care funding and demand for healthcare. Given the insufficient number of GPs, recruitment is difficult and they are expensive to employ. Although recently prioritised for investment, primary care funding had previously been falling in real terms for years, despite increasing workload. Demand from an older, increasingly complex population is ever-rising. With inadequate availability, limited funding and growing demand, it makes sense to use GPs where their expertise is best utilised; seeing complex conditions, managing complicated risk and dealing with multimorbidity. Minor illness, and indeed chronic diseases such as asthma, high blood pressure and diabetes, are increasingly the domain of the specialised practice nurse, supported by a GP if necessary.

'Traditional' GP practices, where such changes have yet to occur, are disappearing. The days of lone GP partners seeing everything from minor illness to chronic disease to complex cases are gone – such an approach seems unsustainable, both financially and for effectively managing demand. These practices either close or adapt; it appears that pursuing the latter approach too late may lead to the former becoming more likely.

However, recruiting practice nurses also tends to be difficult. There have long been too few to meet demand, and various recent developments, including Brexit, seem to have further negatively impacted nursing registrations and applications. The widespread understanding that practice nurses allow for more sustainable primary care has meant even greater demand for these professionals and exacerbated the challenges in recruiting them.

Government plans to enhance GP and nurse numbers are well publicised, but even if the most ambitious projections are realised, recruitment may still be insufficient to allow continuation of our current way of working. It is therefore recognised that we must look to professions other than doctors and nurses to provide much-needed clinical capacity in primary care.

Joining the traditional workforce are newer additions to the general practice team. The training of physician associates has expanded dramatically in recent years, and paramedics are increasingly working in primary care. With appropriate training, both these professional groups are well suited to managing minor illness. Most notable in numbers, however, is the advent of practice-based clinical pharmacists.

In contrast to the recruitment difficulties for doctors and nurses, there exists a relative surplus of highly trained pharmacists. These health professionals, many of whom can prescribe and are already experienced in minor illness management, are increasingly leaving pharmacies to work in GP practices. This movement appears further accelerated by recent funding changes for community pharmacies and has been apparent in courses run by the National Minor Illness Centre (NMIC) – attended by just a few pharmacists in previous years but with whole courses filled by pharmacists more recently.

There is substantial backing for this change. NHS England's *General Practice Forward View*, published in 2016, expressly endorses the expansion of workforce capacity with physician associates and clinical pharmacists. This is accompanied by considerable central investment and an expectation for local health economies to facilitate such recruitment.

In the coming years, skill mix in primary care will likely broaden accordingly. Along with nurses, clinical pharmacists, physician associates and paramedics, we are also likely to see in-house physiotherapists and mental health professionals. Given the proportion of primary care capacity spent managing musculoskeletal issues and mental health conditions, such further additions to the team seem entirely sensible.

Concerns that patients may react unfavourably to these changes are, in the view of the authors, likely overplayed. Though people often speak fondly of the days when GPs were available for face-to-face advice, medically related or not, at a moment's notice regardless of non-urgency, most recognise that this is simply no longer feasible. Given current challenges in capacity, people's expectations increasingly relate to just being able to access care with someone suitably skilled within an appropriate time frame.

It is important to note that, as well as enhancing financial viability, aiding workforce recruitment and reducing unmet demand, diversifying skill mix will likely provide additional quality benefits. A multitude of different professions working together encourages learning from each other's diverse backgrounds, experience and expertise, while allowing optimal utilisation of each profession's individual strengths. Compared with a GP, a physiotherapist may excel in assessing and treating musculoskeletal issues, while a pharmacist may be more effective in medication reviews and improving concordance. The diversity makes the team more effective overall, while also enhancing efficiency and sustainability.

The care quality benefits may also extend outside the walls of GP practices. Recognising that practice-based allied health professionals often pursue portfolio careers, working part-time in their more conventional roles, their performance in each setting can be enhanced by the other.

Emergency care practitioner paramedics who undergo training in minor illness management and gain clinical experience in primary care are likely to be more effective in their role as ambulance paramedics responding to 999 calls. Despite the urgency suggested by the context, much of the pressure facing ambulances comes from self-limiting or minor illness, for which traditional paramedic training is arguably lacking. The dual role across settings may allow for such cases to avoid conveyance to hospital, saving scarce healthcare resources while providing more appropriate care to people in their own homes.

Similarly, pharmacists can transfer the skills and experience gained in GP settings into community pharmacy services. Minor ailments schemes and medication use reviews have existed for years in community pharmacy, helping to reduce pressure on GP practices, but chronic disease management in pharmacies is relatively novel. The detection of high blood pressure, initiation of medication and titration to target is already occurring in some community pharmacies; more clinical pathways are likely to follow. Proficiency in consultation skills and shared decision-making is invaluable for moving such work into community pharmacy, with resultant benefits for patients, GP practices and participating pharmacies.

HOW CARE IS GIVEN

In response to the pressures faced by the NHS, our ways of working need to adapt. Areas of inefficiency, such as the communication channels between primary, community, secondary and social care, undoubtedly need to improve further. Minor illness management and our approach to treating infectious diseases is very likely to change, given increasing antibiotic resistance. Technology will allow new forms of interaction, with new opportunities and new challenges, likely underpinned by an emphasis on prevention and self-care; this will be essential for meeting demand and curbing its growth. In this section, we will review these different areas and how minor illness management seems likely to evolve, albeit with the caveat that new 'disruptive technology', by its very nature, may lead to developments hitherto unforeseen.

Our current channels for interprofessional communication have a tendency to invoke confusion and disbelief. Patients and clinicians alike, quite reasonably, cannot understand why communication between NHS organisations in the 21st century often still relies on the receipt of letters (whether by post or electronically). Questions frequently posed include: 'Why don't we all write into the same record?', 'Why can't we access the results of tests others have organised?' and 'Why isn't the communication instant?'

Such inefficiencies deplete scarce capacity that could be otherwise employed in directly providing care. Behind the scenes, however, change is happening. The shared care record is expanding in scope, and local health economies are investing into enhancing system interoperability across primary, community and secondary care. Though it has been long in the making, within the next few years, we should see a transformation in digital health records: owned, controlled and accessible by the patient.

Any pessimism here would be understandable – indeed, the failure of previous high profile, and very expensive, information technology (IT) endeavours are painfully memorable. If doubts persist despite NHS IT infrastructure being highlighted as a priority following the cyberattack in 2017, optimism may be derived from the tangible progress observed by *The Minor Illness Manual*'s authors through their patient encounters.

In the past few years, the number of services inputting into the patient record accessed by primary care has progressively expanded. Contacts with out-of-hours care, dietitians, district nurses, community matrons, the musculoskeletal clinic, community chronic disease services and social care, spanning multiple organisations, are becoming effortlessly visible to primary care (although navigating the morass of detail may be increasingly difficult). Newly commissioned services are often mandated to input into the primary care system; this list will likely continue to grow as existing contracts come to term and are re-tendered. This is in stark contrast to the situation just a few years ago, when no encounters outside the GP practice were directly visible in the primary care record.

Minor illness management has directly benefitted from this; access to examination findings and recorded vital signs from an out-of-hours consultation allows illness trajectory to be tracked. If the patient later presents to the GP practice, such trends are extremely useful in establishing context and thereby assessing risk. An example would be someone presenting with a cough. Oxygen saturations of 96% with mildly reduced air entry are less concerning in the context of having risen from 94% a few days previously and crepitations having cleared than if saturations were 98% a few days previously with no chest signs.

The notable omission in the parties inputting into a shared record tends to be the local hospital. Primary care's inability to see an account of outpatient appointments until a clinic letter is received weeks later is an ongoing source of inefficiency and frustration. However, given the progress made thus far, the potential benefits of remedying these processes, and the clear commitment expressed across the system, it seems likely that a shared care record will soon follow. The additional workload and problematic delay arising from letter-based communication and poorly interoperable systems will then join handwritten prescriptions and paper pathology requests in representing the inefficiencies of a bygone era.

The sharing of medical records is merely one element of how technology will transform the way in which we work. Though more specific predictions here would be unwise, and indeed the most revolutionary developments may be largely unexpected, it is probably safe to say that we will see pioneering innovation with new investigations and treatments. One area where such development is crucially needed is to address the increasing problem of antimicrobial resistance.

Resistance to antibiotics is one of the greatest challenges facing modern healthcare and, despite current efforts at stewardship, seems likely to worsen. The recent advent of untreatable infections is a worrying harbinger of problems to come; without effective antibiotics, surgery and chemotherapy could become prohibitively risky, while mortality from common infectious diseases could rise to levels yet unseen in the modern world. New commercial models with the pharmaceutical industry are currently under discussion to incentivise the discovery of novel antimicrobials, with 'old antimicrobials' also being reintroduced to clinical practice.

The global response to antimicrobial resistance, according to the World Health Organization (WHO), will need to be multipronged and target agriculture, animal health and human health. As a major source of antibiotic usage in the latter category, our approach to minor illness management needs to change. Increased vigilance in antibiotic prescribing, with narrow-spectrum agents used preferentially, and greater emphasis on education, self-care and the efficacy of most people's immune systems will be necessary. Remember, even bacterial infections may not need antibiotics and can be mild and self-limiting.

Technology can help in identifying who really needs antibiotics and then appropriately selecting which antibiotics to prescribe. Point-of-care fingerprick blood tests for the inflammatory marker C-reactive protein are already used in some GP practices to assess the need for antibiotic therapy, while rapid antibiotic susceptibility tests are a focus for current research. Reducing inappropriate antibiotic use is very likely to see greater emphasis in the near future; it is even feasible that all minor illness practitioners will be required to have access to point-of-care testing to guide antibiotic therapy, just as a thermometer and stethoscope are currently standard equipment.

The need for point-of-care testing, or at the very least, findings from clinical examination to guide appropriate antibiotic use appears mutually exclusive with another growing trend; the use of e-consultations and video consultations. It is likely that both may see increasing use but in different clinical contexts.

Like telephone consultations, e-consultations and video consultations may have greatest utility in following up people already seen face-to-face or in managing chronic disease, with the patient supplying their own data for the metric to be monitored (such as blood pressure or blood glucose readings). This could even be automated, with consultations only occurring if readings fall outside of defined parameters or if data trends suggest worsening control. However, care must be taken to ensure that our enthusiasm for these new types of consultation does not lead to a two-tier system that disadvantages those who are not comfortable with, or cannot afford, smartphones or Internet access.

While safe and effective assessment of most minor illnesses may necessitate a clinical examination, this could be accomplished remotely in certain situations. After the history has been taken (on the phone or online), someone with a rash, supplying readings of their vital signs and appropriate high-resolution images, could provide a clinician with most of the information available from a traditional examination but without the typical inconvenience associated with seeking care. Likewise, observation of the tonsils would be possible remotely, and with the ubiquity of smartphones, perhaps even remote chest auscultation might become commonplace.

Other technological innovations bundled alongside e-consultations, such as artificial intelligence (AI), are more controversial. AI-driven triage has been trialled in parts of the United Kingdom to support 111, the conventional route for out-of-hours urgent care. Given that 111 call handlers are non-clinical and follow a decision tree, using AI in these circumstances does not seem overly radical. More concerning, however, is the notion of AI chatbots replacing consultations with clinicians.

Making a diagnosis and managing an illness can rely on nuances. People may overplay or underplay their symptoms and express non-verbal cues. Their motivations for seeking help may surprise, and their experience of their symptoms may not match textbook disease profiles. Management requires exploration of health beliefs, tailored discussion to suit individual requirements and negotiation of mutually acceptable options. It is unclear how an AI chatbot would function here.

There is also much more to a consultation than arriving at a diagnosis and generating a management plan. Particularly in minor illness management, the most important aspects can be empathy, compassion and providing someone with reassurance and confidence that their issue, which may seem extremely worrying to them, will resolve on its own with time. It therefore seems unlikely that AI chatbots will replace conventional clinicians in the near future, although we may see their increasing use in protocol-driven triage and pre-consultation information gathering.

Given the challenges posed by rising demand and the resultant pressures on the health service, use of technology in these ways is likely to aid sustainability. However, this alone will probably not be enough. As well as meeting demand through technology, it will be essential to focus on reducing the demand itself, or at least curbing its increase. Our clinical interactions are key to this. Every encounter is an opportunity to guide behaviour change, to explore health-seeking behaviour, and through understanding underlying beliefs, motivators, concerns and expectations, appropriately educate people to better care for themselves. The Internet is already democratising healthcare; we must further leverage this to our advantage in promoting better self-management while taking care to avoid cyberchondria.

Modern media and technology have an important role in mass education, as seen with antibiotic stewardship, but the individualised education and feedback given in each consultation is invaluable. Knowing when to seek medical attention, the typical duration of a minor illness, how to self-care, and where such advice can be accessed (e.g. online at NHS Choices or through local community pharmacies) are critical to modifying inappropriate health-seeking behaviour and freeing up capacity for the people needing it most.

This approach extends to chronic conditions. Empowering people in self-management is not only more powerful than an external focus of care dependent on health professionals, but also reduces pressure on the system overall. Greater emphasis on patient-centred approaches such as motivational interviewing and health coaching could have the transformative potential to shift the locus of responsibility from the system to the individual, combining enhanced effectiveness with fewer side effects than conventional medical management.

Despite (and due to) the financial challenges facing the system, greater investment in disease prevention and proactive care will be necessary. Confined by the limitations conferred by one-year financial cycles, local health economies have tended to prioritise short-term measures over long-term preventative strategies. Although the latter may take years to deliver savings, thus making the case for such spending difficult in an uncertain financial climate, the funding of disease prevention will be essential for future sustainability.

Investment in prevention and general wellbeing can lead to impressive dividends, far outweighing the initial outlay. The incidence of cardiovascular disease, type 2 diabetes and some cancers is linked to unhealthy diets, physical inactivity and obesity, all of which also increase susceptibility to infection and minor illness. The connection with lifestyle extends beyond physical measures of wellbeing; feeling stressed or unhappy similarly inhibits the immune system. Much of the demand currently challenging primary care, and predicted to further grow, could be avoided with greater proactive focus on people keeping well and following a healthy, balanced and less sedentary lifestyle.

If preventing pathology is unsuccessful, early intervention still tends to offer much better value than treating well-established pathology. Resourcing the identification and more effective management of high blood pressure would likely pay for itself through fewer heart attacks and strokes; more intensively managing newly-diagnosed type 2 diabetes (without inflicting hypoglycaemia), would likely attenuate the rise in spend on diabetes complications (roughly 80% of the £10 billion spent annually in the NHS on diabetes is attributable to the complications of the disease).

In addition to the obvious human benefits of keeping people happier and healthier, the business case for prevention and proactive care is undeniable. Recent NHS strategy would seem to agree, having invested millions of pounds in the world's first nationwide intervention to prevent type 2 diabetes. As healthcare demand continues to outpace resource availability, initiatives such as the NHS Diabetes Prevention Programme, aimed at encouraging people to take control of their health and promoting lasting behaviour change, will become ever more important in enhancing the sustainability of our system.

HOW CARE IS ORGANISED

If attempting to predict future technology is unwise, there is arguably little hope for accurately predicting future NHS structures. Nonetheless, the organisation of our healthcare system warrants examination as the changes underway are likely to have practical repercussions for all healthcare practitioners. In this section, we will therefore look at the direction of travel for primary care and the internal mechanisms of the NHS, as well as the reasoning underlying Sustainability and Transformation Partnerships (STPs) and Integrated Care Systems (ICSs). Given the current pace of change, it should be noted that, while accurate at the time of publication, the information here is particularly prone to becoming obsolete.

The traditional model of primary care with multiple, independent GP practices is becoming progressively less viable. The combination of increasing workload, difficulty recruiting and challenging finances is, as you might expect, untenable. Small, stand-alone practices tend to be more fragile; an unforeseen problem, such as a GP becoming sick, can push these practices into a descending spiral of financial difficulty, burnout and eventual closure.

This is not just theoretical; over 250 GP practices closed or merged in 2017/18, with the vast majority being smaller practices (the average list size of these practices was 3887 – around half of the average list size for all GP practices in England). Merging, where possible, is almost invariably preferable to closure, and not just for the patients. One practice collapsing may trigger a domino effect; surrounding practices, themselves with overstretched staff, struggle to accommodate the dispersed patients and may become unsustainably overwhelmed and demoralised, destabilising local primary care.

There is safety in numbers. The enhanced resilience made possible through being larger has seen mergers between practices at an unprecedented scale. These 'super-practices' may have hundreds of GP partners and serve hundreds of thousands of registered patients; compared to the small, stand-alone practice, the impact of a GP becoming sick is negligible.

Such size offers many other potential benefits. Buying at scale means cheaper supplies than multiple small organisations buying separately from different suppliers. Greater efficiency can arise through sharing 'back office' functions such as secretarial provision, human resources and payroll. Diversifying skill mix is facilitated through having enough demand to justify the aforementioned physiotherapist or having sufficient home visit requests to warrant an emergency care practitioner paramedic.

Though often cited as a concern with large practices, continuity of care need not suffer. Each GP can maintain their own list and keep oversight over their patients' care, even if the care itself comes from other members of the team. Indeed, the quality of care can benefit from opportunities afforded by such size. The workforce may be large enough to allow for a variety of in-house specialist expertise – rather than waiting months for a hospital dermatology or gynaecology appointment, people may instead see a specialist GP in the practice without delay. Services that smaller practices may struggle to provide, such as 24-hour electrocardiograms (ECGs), minor surgery, or extended access, are more feasible with greater size and may benefit the practice as well as its patients through providing additional revenue.

Mergers and federations are not a prerequisite for collaboration. Many practices are adopting more informal arrangements by remaining as separate entities but sharing staff (such as clinical pharmacists) across sites or providing cross-cover. Whichever form it takes, working together serves to support practices' resilience and thereby enhance local primary care stability.

With encouragement from both NHS England and Local Medical Committees, we are likely to see greater collaboration still. The future model of primary care will not feature multiple, independent GP practices but a more united body, regardless of the contractual ties between parts.

Practitioners of minor illness can expect more dynamic working arrangements, perhaps delivering care across multiple practices or in primary care hubs resourced by the practices served. Referrals to specialist colleagues, such as a diabetes specialist nurse in a neighbouring practice or a physiotherapist in another, may become commonplace, with greater convenience for the patient, reduced delay and care closer to home. Importantly, work may also feel less lonely than at present; being part of a large, well-functioning team can greatly enhance job satisfaction while providing varied opportunities for professional growth and development.

The changes taking place in the organisation of care extend beyond GP practices. Wider healthcare systems are evolving in form and structure, with long-established relationships and patterns of behaviour between constituent organisations undergoing reform. Though representing perhaps the most exciting change to the NHS in recent memory, it is appreciated that not everyone would be enthralled by a detailed explanation of STPs and ICSs. We shall, therefore, attempt to navigate this area relatively swiftly and succinctly, while explaining these commonly heard acronyms and providing insight into the complex revolution taking place.

As is often the case with understanding reorganisation, a useful starting point is to examine the flow of resources. Even those with many years of NHS service may have little appreciation of the underlying payment mechanisms in its internal market, let alone the inequity between primary and secondary care. The costs of care have seldom been communicated to front-line staff, particularly in hospital settings. If unaware yourself, ask a colleague for the rough price of an A&E attendance/admission/outpatient appointment locally.

The reality might surprise you. At the time of publication, a first outpatient appointment is charged at roughly the same price as a year of care from a GP practice. Perhaps take a moment to process that. A single outpatient appointment with a specialist (who may be a junior doctor supported by a consultant) costs the system roughly the same as the near-limitless encounters someone may have with their GP practice, including home visits, over an entire year. Surprised?

Yet, if hospital-based care is so expensive, why does so much work still occur there? Unlike GP practices, where a relatively fixed sum is paid per patient per year regardless of how many appointments they need, contracts for hospitals are generally activity-based. This means that each A&E attendance, emergency admission, surgical procedure and outpatient appointment is invoiced (according to tariff) to the local commissioners. However, unlike most situations where a bill must be paid, those paying the bill here have limited control over what has been ordered.

GP referrals and the manner in which their population seeks healthcare are the main drivers and deciders of commissioners' spending. Everyone presenting to A&E with a minor illness results in additional avoidable expenditure, reducing the resources available for investment in prevention, community services and primary care, thus further impacting the capacity for these services to meet growing demand. This clearly lends itself to a vicious cycle with overburdened primary care driving expensive hospital activity and stripping away potential financial support.

This payment system may also pre-dispose to antagonism between commissioners and providers rather than collaboration. Reliant on income secured through activity (i.e. the number of times people are seen), hospitals are generally not incentivised to reduce contact. Combined with their ability to generate additional activity such as follow-up appointments, it would perhaps be unsurprising if more appointments might occur than absolutely necessary.

Meanwhile, the commissioners, with a set budget and statutory duty not to overspend, endeavour to reduce avoidable hospital activity. In the quest for avoiding overspending, local hospitals, as the main areas of expenditure, tend to represent commissioners' obvious targets for financial efficiencies. Initiatives to reduce activity, such as contracting with external providers for cheaper elective surgery, can then destabilise the hospitals. The external providers may undercut hospital tariffs through cherry-picking less complex patients, not hosting intensive care facilities and not seeing emergencies. The hospitals, however, must provide for all and must make up for lost income.

The result can be a perpetual cat-and-mouse game with the hospitals and the commissioners trying hard to achieve a financial outcome that is inherently detrimental to the other. Despite drawing inordinate effort from all parties, the dynamics resulting from activity-based-tariff contracts may do little to improve care and, as collateral damage, may fuel the resource inequity affecting GP practices. There is increasing recognition of this; STPs and ICSs are part of the response.

The first step in changing relationships was unsurprisingly to encourage communication. In late 2015, NHS planning guidance first mentioned STPs, requiring areas that may have previously worked completely separately to start working together as a geography. There were 44 STPs in total across England; in each, all the commissioners, comprising clinical commissioning groups and local authorities, and all the providers, including hospitals, ambulance services, mental health services, community care providers and GP practices, were expected to work together to enhance sustainability.

This word, 'sustainability', has been unfairly labelled by some as a euphemism for 'cutting services'. Whilst it is certainly true that the STPs are tasked with generating efficiencies, in the context of an NHS budget shortfall in the order of billions of pounds, this would seem essential and entirely sensible. Though some STPs, based on local need and circumstances, may decommission some services in pursuit of securing optimal value for taxpayer money, STPs are generally likely to create many more services in the community, with more convenient and accessible care delivered closer to people's homes, driven by commissioning for outcomes rather than processes.

The natural evolution of STP collaboration is the ICS. Put simply, an ICS acknowledges that an area's funding is fixed, and all organisations must work within its financial confines to provide care to the whole population. The financial health of the whole system is important so it is in everyone's interests to work together. Payment structures may change accordingly; instead of being paid on activity, hospitals might receive a lump sum for all the care provided to the population, much like GP practices. Significant cultural shifts and behaviour changes are then likely to follow.

With additional activity no longer driving income but instead increasing pressure on services, hospitals are unlikely to welcome such activity and may be more inclined to work to strengthen primary and community care to reduce attendances, admissions and referrals. All organisations would thus have aligned incentives and would be motivated to provide care in the most efficient and effective manner available, regardless of the building. Aspects of this vision are reminiscent of the NHS before the internal market was introduced in 1991, when the National Health Service provided healthcare to the nation and gave less attention to which part of its budget was financially responsible for each event.

Where prevention of disease had previously been regarded as mostly a primary care and public health issue, hospitals would now seek active involvement in optimising prevention and reducing demand for their services. Where face to face appointments previously predominated in hospitals (and attracted greater tariff), consultants would now be encouraged to conduct appropriate appointments remotely, with greater convenience for all. Where hospitals and commissioners may have previously held opposing interests, both would now collaborate to improve efficiency and redirect efforts towards enhancing population health. Compared with our current systems, it may be a revolution in approach and thinking.

Clinicians working in ICSs may be redeployed across organisations. The diabetes consultant may see hospital inpatients, run community clinics and, rather than only seeing referrals, proactively search primary care systems for people warranting review. Such an approach greatly assists in appropriate and timely intensification of treatment and supporting the population to avoid disease complications. Likewise, minor illness practitioners may work across collaborating practices and, broader still, across an alliance of providers including community services and local hospitals. The benefits of a workforce shared across urgent care clinics, community admission avoidance services and hospital A&E departments are clear, both for consistency in the approach to care and for up-skilling the workforce themselves.

Although a mere glimpse into how the NHS is evolving, we hope that this chapter has provided sufficient insight into the changes in motion regarding who delivers care, how it is given and how it is organised, to allow you to share our enthusiasm about its future. Necessity is the mother of invention; with staying the same simply not an option, the pressures on our health system are forcing it to develop in new and very exciting ways.

The elements in this complex structure are finally coming into alignment, sharing an ethos of sustainable, population-based management of health and wellbeing. With disparate financial motivations largely nullified, the whole system is moving together to deliver the right care in the right place at the right time, while striving to use resources wisely to achieve maximal benefit.

Armed with a diverse, flexible and dedicated workforce, and embracing the opportunities of technology and population empowerment in facing its challenges, the NHS is rallying to ensure not only survival but to surpass current standards and remain the best healthcare system worldwide.

Indeed, the NHS of the future, somewhat ironically, seems to match its original blueprint: a united system, unconcerned with internal financial transactions and equitably centred on high-quality care for all. Although admittedly oversimplified, 70 years after the launch of NHS, we appear in some ways to be arriving back at the start. Now, who said its changes aren't cyclical?

CHAPTER 2

Introduction

GENERAL ADVICE

History

- Listening is the greatest skill. What is the patient's agenda?
- Open questions may reveal hidden concerns
- Most diagnoses are made on the history – 'Listen to the patient: they are telling you the diagnosis'

Examination

- This may reveal important signs but will also serve to reassure the patient
- It invades the patient's personal space – be sensitive to this

Tests

- Not usually helpful in minor illness
- Only useful if the management depends on the result
- May give false-positive results and cause unnecessary concern
- May be misleading – for example, by identifying bacteria that are harmless commensals

Self-care

- Discuss the options and agree the proposed plan of management with the patient
- For a choice to be genuine, the patient needs to be informed about the options
- Worsening advice: explain the likely progress and ask the patient to contact the most appropriate NHS service if the situation worsens or there is no improvement within a specified time
- Handouts may be useful, for example, patient.info, *When Should I Worry* leaflet or TARGET toolkit (see References)

Prescription

- Always check with the current British National Formulary (BNF) or British National Formulary for Children (BNFC)
- Be aware of local guidelines, as patterns of antibiotic resistance vary nationally

Caution

- Although guidelines support clinical judgement, they can never replace experience and intuition. If you feel concerned about the patient, always seek advice
- Be aware of the unique limits of your own competence and never exceed them
- Be alert for red flags

 RED FLAGS

Red flags are factors that suggest a serious condition rather than a minor illness. Unless you are very experienced, the presence of a red flag requires referral of the patient to a senior colleague. To help you to decide on the best course of action, which depends on your expertise and place of work, we have given a brief indication of the possible serious diagnosis and appropriate management. We are aware that some of the suggested pathways can currently only be accessed via a doctor. We also recognise the challenge of finding the best course of action for a patient who is remotely assessed. A patient requiring urgent assessment in a hospital setting will encounter additional delay through attending A&E compared with a direct referral to a specialty by the assessing clinician, as well as incurring additional expense for the health system. However, in exceptional circumstances, there may not be another feasible option.

HIGH-RISK GROUPS FOR INFECTIONS

Immunosuppressed

- Due to *medication*: for example, prednisolone, azathioprine, disease-modifying antirheumatic drugs (DMARDs) such as methotrexate, antithyroid drugs such as carbimazole, ciclosporin, cyclophosphamide, chemotherapy (and up to 6 months after), also non-steroidal anti-inflammatory drugs (NSAIDs; weak immunosuppressant action that increases risk of secondary infections where the skin is not intact)
- Due to *medical conditions* that reduce the immune response. These include human immunodeficiency virus (HIV), leukaemia, lymphoma, neutropenia, splenectomy, sickle cell anaemia, malnutrition, pregnancy, prematurity (up to the age of 2), inherited immunodeficiency and most commonly diabetes, especially if poorly controlled (Box 2.1). For information on checking for suspected diabetes, see Chapter 8

BOX 2.1   PATIENTS WITH DIABETES

Poorly controlled diabetes makes the patient immunosuppressed, but even if the diabetes is normally well controlled, infection may cause hyperglycaemia, which acutely impairs the immune response and risks tipping the patient into diabetic ketoacidosis. All patients with diabetes should have a care plan that tells them what to do if they are unwell. The details will vary, but the principles are:

- Don't reduce your insulin or tablets just because you are not eating much
- Keep eating as much as you are able. If you are unable to eat, drink something nutritious
- Have lots of sugar-free drinks
- If you think you are becoming dehydrated, seek help immediately
- If you test your blood glucose levels, do so more frequently, and check for ketones if your blood glucose is above 17 mmol/L or you feel very thirsty or breathless

---

Long-term conditions

- Significant heart, lung, kidney, liver or neuromuscular disease

MEDICATION ADVICE

Dose of medication

The appropriate adult dose of medication for a condition is given in the text of this book. For the latest information, see the BNF and, for children, the BNFC.

Risk alerts for medications

The table that follows lists abbreviations found after drug names in the text where there is a significant risk of adverse events. Any drug may have potential for multiple interactions, but the majority are not clinically significant. The tags provide warnings where there is a risk. Manufacturers often advise against the use of a medication in pregnancy or breastfeeding when there is insufficient evidence of safety. Independent information sources, such as the BNF, UK Teratology Information Service (UKTIS) and Drugs and Lactation Database (LactMed) may advise that there is no evidence of harm. A balance needs to be struck to avoid denying pregnant or lactating women helpful medication whilst maintaining adequate safety for the foetus or infant.

The tags to each drug name may vary depending on the context. For example, oral prednisolone is suitable for use in asthma for a pregnant woman where the benefit outweighs the risk, but not when it is being considered as an option to treat hay fever.

It should be remembered that the elimination of many drugs can be affected by renal or hepatic impairment. If the patient has either, check the dose of the drug in the relevant section of the BNF/BNFC.

These symbols are designed to alert you quickly and simply to prescribing issues which are common and important (Table 2.1). They cannot cover all possibilities; full information on prescribing is available in the BNF and BNFC.

Table 2.1 Prescribing symbols used in this book

P	**Pregnancy** risk. Use an alternative medication known to be safe in pregnancy. If the patient is allergic to penicillin, alternatives include cefalexin or erythromycin. Cefalexin, which shares some molecular structure with penicillins, should not be used if the patient has had an anaphylactic reaction to any penicillin. Erythromycin is preferred to clarithromycin if a macrolide is needed. Information sources: BNF or UKTIS.
B	**Breastfeeding** risk. The drug affects breastfeeding or is secreted in milk and is not suitable for the baby. Use an alternative medication known to be safe in breastfeeding. Information sources: BNF or LactMed.
C	**Children**. The medication is either harmful to children or has a limited licence; for example, the medicine may only be licensed for children over a certain age. Information source: BNFC.
I	**Interactions** likely. For example, macrolides such as clarithromycin inhibit the liver enzymes that metabolise drugs. This can result in an accumulation of another drug to potentially toxic levels. Many drugs can be affected (e.g., amlodipine, colchicine, simvastatin, ticagrelor and warfarin), so always check the BNF for any interaction before prescribing. If a macrolide is needed but clarithromycin is precluded because of interactions, consider azithromycin, which does not interact significantly with the hepatic cytochrome P450 system. Information sources: BNF or EMC.
Q	**QT interval** prolonged. Avoid for anyone with a known long QT interval, an unknown QT interval plus a family history of unexplained sudden death, or for anyone already taking another drug that prolongs the interval. A long interval between the Q and T waves on an ECG indicates an increased risk of cardiac arrhythmias that can cause sudden death. Information sources: SADS or CredibleMeds.

Websites
BNF: bnf.nice.org.uk
BNFC: bnfc.nice.org.uk
CredibleMeds: www.crediblemeds.org
EMC: www.medicines.org.uk
LactMed: toxnet.nlm.nih.gov/newtoxnet/lactmed.htm
SADS: www.sads.org.uk
UKTIS: www.uktis.org

References

Patient Info. https://patient.info/
Royal College of General Practitioners (RCGP). 2017. TARGET antibiotic toolkit. www.rcgp.org.uk/TARGETantibiotics
When Should I Worry. www.whenshouldiworry.com. *A booklet for parents about respiratory tract infections in children.*

CHAPTER 3

Fever and sepsis

FEVERISH ILLNESS

Sometimes fever alone is the presenting problem. In UK primary care, this is more likely to be due to viral than bacterial infection. A careful history can usually identify the likely source, but sometimes this is not obvious. Be aware that although most patients with a flu-like illness may indeed have a simple viral infection, there are many uncommon diseases that can cause the same initial symptoms. Ask open questions to see if there could be an alternative source of infection (such as the urinary tract). This is particularly important if the history has some odd features, or if the symptoms have been present for more than 5 days. Fever in children is considered separately later in this chapter.

RED FLAGS

SEPSIS

Sepsis is 'life-threatening organ dysfunction due to a dysregulated host response to infection'. It is underrecognised in primary care and it has a high mortality. Many of the 'red flags' for different conditions indicate a risk of sepsis. For more information, see the NICE guideline NG51 (2016) and the Sepsis Toolkit of the Royal College of General Practitioners (RCGP 2016).

Consider sepsis if the patient appears very unwell. Fever is usually present, but the very young, old or frail patients may have a normal temperature. Low temperature ≤36°C and/or drowsiness are also warning signs, especially if there are risk factors for sepsis:

- Under 1 year or over 75 years of age
- Frailty
- Immunosuppression (see previous chapter)
- Surgery or other invasive procedure in past 6 weeks
- Pregnancy (or recent termination/miscarriage)
- Breach of skin (e.g. cuts, burns or skin infections)
- Intravenous drug misuse
- Indwelling lines or catheters

History

- Duration
- Joint and muscle pains, especially leg pain in children and young people (Thompson et al., 2006)
- Sore throat
- Headache
- Sneezing/nasal discharge
- Cough – productive?
- Rash
- Vomiting/diarrhoea
- Abdominal pain
- ⚑ Photophobia
- ⚑ Drowsiness
- ⚑ Urinary symptoms
- ⚑ Rigors/shaking (suggest bacterial infection)
- ⚑ Prostration (unable to stand up, difficulty in walking)
- ⚑ Pregnancy
- ⚑ Lactating

🏳 Travel to tropical region in last 12 months

🏳 Exposure to rats' urine (e.g. in sewers or rivers)

🏳 Recent operation, bites or cuts

🏳 High-risk group (see Chapter 2)

Examination (modified as suggested by symptoms)

- Mental state – drowsiness?
- Temperature (taking into account any recent antipyretic)
- Pulse rate
- Respiratory rate
- Blood pressure in adults, capillary refill time (CRT) in children
- Oxygen saturation, if respiratory infection or sepsis is suspected
- Hydration
- Ears
- Throat
- Cervical lymph nodes
- Chest (auscultation and percussion)
- Any rash (if so, does it blanch?)
- Any wounds or breaks in skin
- If no focus of infection is found, look carefully for a rash and test the urine
- If meningitis is suspected, look for restriction of neck or back movement (e.g. can a child kiss his knees?)
- Gait and coordination
- In a lactating woman, check the breasts
- Examine any painful area (e.g. abdomen)

Tests

- If the cause of fever is not obvious, test urine for nitrites, leucocytes, blood and glucose (to avoid contaminating the whole sample, pour a little urine on the test strip). If using bottles containing boric acid, make sure that your test strip is compatible
- Send midstream urine (MSU) for culture in a feverish patient if test positive or any urinary symptoms
- Consider blood glucose (in a patient without diabetes, a blood glucose >7.7 mmol/L may indicate sepsis)
- If travel to tropical area in last 12 months, consider sending thick and thin blood film for malaria and full blood count (FBC). If the first test is negative, repeat the blood film after 12 to 24 hours. If the second test is negative, repeat the blood film again after a further 24 hours

Self-care

- Assume a viral cause if no other clues, fever less than 5 days' duration and generally well
- Otherwise give treatment appropriate to the cause
- Adequate fluid intake
- Avoid over-strenuous activity
- Reduce anxiety about fever by explaining that it is produced by the body in response to an infection to boost the effective immune response. Fever itself does not cause any harm, and may aid recovery. It is important to make parents and patients aware that the fever caused by an infection is not dangerous but is 'a sign that the immune system is busy'
- There is no evidence that antipyretic medicines can prevent febrile convulsions (NICE, 2013), and we do not yet know whether their use may delay recovery from infection (Drewry et al., 2017). See the references that follow for evidence that:
  - Antipyretic use increased mortality in animals with influenza (Eyers et al., 2010)
  - The replication of meningococci is reduced at high temperatures (Dixon et al., 2010)
  - Paracetamol reduces the immune response to vaccination (Prymula et al., 2014)
  - The distress of an unwell child may be unrelated to the fever (Corrard et al., 2017)

- Suppressing fever may increase the spread of infection (Earn et al., 2014)
  - The aim of giving an antipyretic should be to improved child's overall comfort rather than focusing on the normalisation of body temperature (Sullivan et al., 2016)
- Advise on what to do if symptoms worsen; 'worsening advice' or 'safety netting'. Explain the warning signs of sepsis, give a handout, and advise patient to have someone with them who will check them regularly

Prescription

- For a flu-like illness, antiviral medicines (oseltamivir, zanamivir) may be recommended (Public Health England, 2016), but only when the Chief Medical Officer has announced that influenza is circulating in the community (for primary care prescribing). However, in studies, they shortened the duration of the illness by less than 1 day and did not reduce the risk of complications (Heneghan et al., 2016; Ebell et al., 2017). The risk of contracting pneumonia was reduced by 4%, and the risk of being admitted to hospital was reduced by 1%. Prophylactic oseltamivir was associated with a 3% reduction in the absolute risk of laboratory-confirmed influenza (European Centre for Disease Prevention and Control, 2017)
- If antibiotics are indicated, prescribe in line with local resistance patterns (particularly relevant for urinary tract infections)

 RED FLAGS

- Photophobia, drowsiness, neck or back stiffness or non-blanching (petechial) rash (*possible meningitis; dial 999 and give benzylpenicillin IV or IM*)
- Severe illness, rigors, or prostration (unable to stand up) (*likely sepsis; admit to Medical or Paediatrics via 999 ambulance*)
- Urinary symptoms (*likely pyelonephritis or prostatitis; refer to senior colleague*)
- Unexplained fever lasting more than 5 days (*unlikely to be viral; assess for urinary tract infection (UTI) or secondary bacterial infection. In a young child, check for signs of Kawasaki disease*)
- Pregnancy (*consider pyelonephritis and listeriosis. In pregnant women, advise regular paracetamol because there is concern that fever may increase the risk of miscarriage (although randomised controlled trials are lacking and a cohort study did not support this concept; Anderson et al., 2002)*)
- Lactating (*mastitis may cause flu-like symptoms in a breastfeeding woman with only minimal signs in the breast; examine breasts and follow advice in 'Women's Health' section*)
- Travel to tropical area in last 12 months (*malaria or other tropical disease; seek advice*)
- Exposure to rats' urine (*risk of leptospirosis; arrange blood test for serology and consider doxycycline*)
- Neutropenia or current chemotherapy (*probable sepsis; admit immediately*)
- High-risk patient (*high risk of sepsis; seek advice*)
- Dehydration (*admit for IV fluids*)

Action for suspected sepsis

- Dial 999 for an ambulance and use the word 'sepsis'
- Alert the hospital team
- Give high-flow oxygen in adults, if needed, to achieve saturations of at least 94%
- Patients with moderate-to-severe chronic obstructive pulmonary disease (COPD) should have oxygen saturation monitored to achieve 88%–92%
- Give oxygen to children if saturations are ≤90%

FEVERISH ILLNESS IN CHILDREN UNDER FIVE: THE NICE 'TRAFFIC LIGHT' SYSTEM

We recommend that you study the summary of NICE guideline CG160 (revised in 2017), which provides a framework for the assessment of feverish children. There are some differences in the reference ranges for pulse and respiratory rate between this guideline and NG51. We suggest that in this case you follow the advice from NG51, as in Figure 3.1, because it is more recent and more detailed. We would like to draw your attention to the following points:

The routine assessment of a feverish child should always include:

- Temperature (taken with an axillary thermometer in babies under 4 weeks)
- Heart rate
- Respiratory rate
- Capillary refill time

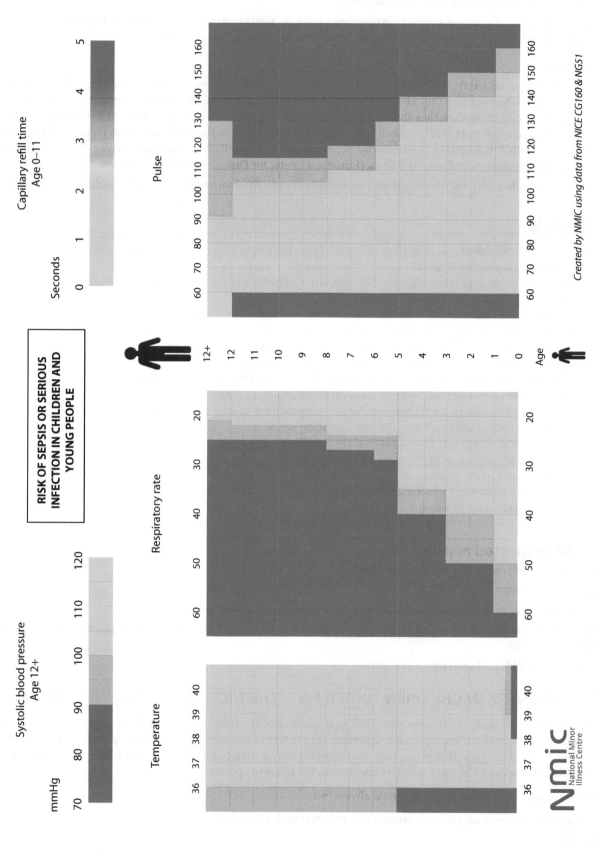

Figure 3.1 Risk of sepsis: pulse and respiratory rate ranges at different ages.

A temperature of ≥38°C in a baby under 3 months is an indication for hospital assessment. However, whether this should apply in the 48 hours after a meningitis B (Men B) vaccination is controversial (Vesikari et al., 2013; NICE, 2017). Our assessment is that most primary care clinicians would not routinely refer a feverish (but otherwise well) baby in the 48 hours following Men B vaccination. However, in the absence of clear advice from NICE, this decision should be taken by a senior clinician. A temperature of ≥39°C in a baby under 6 months may be a sign of sepsis (amber – intermediate risk). Over the age of 6 months, a high fever is not on its own a sign of sepsis, but a low temperature of ≤36°C at any age suggests sepsis. Antipyretic medicine is sometimes given to children by clinicians as a test, because a good response is thought to exclude serious illness. This is a dangerous assumption, and there is no evidence to support it (NICE, 2017; Roland, 2017).

If using remote assessment:

- A child with red features (Table 3.1) should be seen as soon as possible (and certainly within 2 hours)
- A child with amber features should be seen urgently within a few hours

If using face-to-face assessment:

- A child with red features should be admitted for paediatric assessment (unless fever is the only sign in the 48 hours following Men B vaccination; see previous discussion)
- A child with amber features but no obvious diagnosis should be seen by a senior clinician for assessment of the need for admission. If not admitted, careful safety-netting and follow-up should be arranged

Table 3.1 Assessment of the feverish child under five

Traffic light system for identifying risk of serious illness			
	Green – low risk	Amber – intermediate risk	Red – high risk
Colour (of skin, lips or tongue)	• Normal colour	• Pallor reported by parent/carer	• Pale/mottled/ashen/blue
Activity	• Responds normally to social cues • Content/smiles • Stays awake or awakens quickly • Strong normal cry/not crying	• Not responding normally to social cues • No smile • Wakes only with prolonged stimulation • Decreased activity	• No response to social cues • Appears ill to a healthcare professional • Does not wake or if roused does not stay awake • Weak, high-pitched or continuous cry
Respiratory		• Nasal flaring • Tachypnoea: • RR >50 breaths/minute, age 6–12 months • RR >40 breaths/minute, age >12 months • Oxygen saturation ≤95% in air • Crackles in the chest	• Grunting • Tachypnoea: RR >60 breaths/minute • Moderate or severe chest indrawing
Circulation and hydration	• Normal skin and eyes • Moist mucous membranes	• Tachycardia: • >160 beats/minute, age <12 months • >150 beats/minute, age 12–24 months • >140 beats/minute, age 2–5 years • CRT ≥3 seconds • Dry mucous membranes • Poor feeding in infants • Reduced urine output	• Reduced skin turgor
Other	• None of the amber or red symptoms or signs	• Age 3–6 months, temperature ≥39°C • Fever for ≥5 days • Rigors • Swelling of a limb or joint • Non-weight bearing limb/not using an extremity	• Age <3 months, temperature ≥38°C[a] • Non-blanching rash • Bulging fontanelle • Neck stiffness • Status epilepticus • Focal neurological signs • Focal seizures

Source: NICE CG160 (2017).
CRT, capillary refill time; RR, respiratory rate.
[a] Some vaccinations have been found to induce fever in children aged under 3 months.
This traffic light table should be used in conjunction with the recommendations in the NICE guideline on Feverish illness in children.

References

Andersen, A.M.N., Vastrup, P., Wohlfahrt, J., Andersen, P.K., Olsen, J., and Melbye, M. 2002. Fever in pregnancy and risk of fetal death: A cohort study. *The Lancet*; 360(9345):1552–1556.

Corrard, F., Copin, C., Wollner, A., Elbez, A., Derkx, V., Bechet, S., Levy, C., Boucherat, M., and Cohen, R. 2017. Sickness behavior in feverish children is independent of the severity of fever. An observational, multicenter study. *PLOS ONE*. doi: 10.1371/journal. pone.0171670. *The distress of an unwell child may be unrelated to their fever.*

Dixon, G., Booth, C., Price, E., Westran, R., Turner, M., and Klein, N. 2010. Part of beneficial host response? *BMJ*; 340: c450. doi: 10.1136/ bmj.c450. *Reduced meningococcal growth at higher temperatures. Progressive retardation in growth above 37°C was confirmed in author's comment.*

Drewry, A., Ablordeppey, E., Murray, E., Stoll, C., Izadi, S., Dalton, C., Hardi, A., Fowler, S., Fuller, B., and Colditz G. 2017. Antipyretic therapy in critically Ill septic patients: A systematic review and meta-analysis. *Crit Care Med*; 45(5):806–813. *We do not yet know whether antipyretics may delay recovery from severe infection.*

Earn, D., Andrews, P., and Bolker, B. 2014. Population-level effects of suppressing fever. *Proc Biol Sci*; 281(1778):20132570. *Suppressing fever is likely increase the spread of infection, because people feel well enough to go out and mix with others.*

Ebell, M. 2017. WHO downgrades status of oseltamivir. *BMJ*; 358. doi.org/10.1136/bmj.j3266. *The UK government stockpiled oseltamivir at a cost of over £600 m from 2006 to 2014. In 2017 the World Health Organisation (WHO) removed it from their list of essential drugs when unpublished evidence showed that it was ineffective.*

European Centre for disease prevention and control. 2017. Expert opinion on neuraminidase inhibitors for the prevention and treatment of influenza – review of recent systematic reviews and meta-analyses. https://ecdc.europa.eu/en/publications-data/ expert-opinion-neuraminidase-inhibitors-prevention-and-treatment-influenza-review.

Eyers, S., Weatherall, M., Shirtcliffe, P., Perrin, K., and Beasley, R. 2010. The effect on mortality of antipyretics in the treatment of influenza infection: Systematic review and meta-analysis. *J Roy Soc Med*; 103(10):403–411. *Antipyretic use increased mortality in animals with influenza.*

Heneghan, C., Onakpoya, I., Jones, M., Doshi, P., Del Mar, C., Hama, R., Thompson, M. et al. 2016. Neuraminidase inhibitors for influenza: A systematic review and meta-analysis of regulatory and mortality data. *Health Technol Assess*; 20(42):1–242. *No reduction in mortality.*

NICE CG160. 2017. Fever in Under 5s: Assessment and initial management. www.nice.org.uk/guidance/cg160. *This 2013 guidance was revised in 2017 to acknowledge that 'Some vaccinations have been found to induce fever in children aged under 3 months'. Unfortunately no guidance is given about when such a baby (with post-vaccination fever, but no other signs of serious illness) can safely be managed in primary care.*

NICE NG51. 2016. Sepsis: Recognition, diagnosis and early management. www.nice.org.uk/guidance/ng51

Prymula, R., Esposito, S., Zuccotti, G., Xie, F., Toneatto, D., and Kohl, I. 2014. A phase 2 randomized controlled trial of a multicomponent meningococcal serogroup B vaccine (I). Effects of prophylactic paracetamol on immunogenicity and reactogenicity of routine infant vaccines and 4CMen. *Hum Vaccin & Immunother*; 10(7):1993–2004. *Paracetamol reduces the immune response to Men B vaccine, but most babies developed protective levels of antibody.*

Public Health England (PHE). 2017. Influenza: Treatment and prophylaxis using anti-viral agents. www.gov.uk/government/publications/ influenza-treatment-and-prophylaxis-using-anti-viral-agents. *PHE are still recommending the use of antivirals, despite the evidence.*

RCGP. 2016. Sepsis Toolkit. www.rcgp.org.uk/clinical-and-research/toolkits/sepsis-toolkit.aspx

Roland, D., and Snelson, E. 2018. 'So why didn't you think this baby was ill?' Decision-making in acute paediatrics. *Archives of Disease in Childhood-Education and Practice*, doi: 10.1136/archdischild-2017-313199.

Sullivan, J., and Farrar, H. Fever and antipyretic use in children. 2011. *Pediatrics*; 127(3):580–587. *The primary goal of treating the febrile child should be to improve the child's overall comfort rather than focus on the normalization of body temperature.*

Thompson, M., Ninis, N., Perera, R., Mayon-White, R., Phillips, C., Bailey, L., Harnden, A., Mant, D., and Levin, M. 2006. Clinical recognition of meningococcal disease in children and adolescents. *Lancet*; 367(9508):397–403. *A useful overview of the early signs and symptoms of meningococcal infection.*

Vesikari, T., Esposito, S., Prymula, R., Ypma, E., Kohl, I., Toneatto, D., Dull, P., and Kimura, A. 2013. Immunogenicity and safety of an investigational multicomponent, recombinant, meningococcal serogroup B vaccine (4CMenB) administered concomitantly with routine infant and child vaccinations: Results of two randomised trials. *Lancet*; 381(9869):825–835. *Without prophylactic paracetamol, 77% of babies developed a fever after compound vaccination (including Men B) which would be sufficient to trigger admission to hospital under the guidance of NICE CG160. With paracetamol, this percentage dropped to 40%.*

CHAPTER 4

Respiratory tract infections

ACUTE COUGH

History

- Duration
- Dry/productive/wheezy
- Hoarseness
- Colour of sputum, if bloodstained (red or rusty) or frothy
- Fever
- Chest pain (and location)
- Breathlessness
- Previous similar episodes (how treated and what happened)
- Smoking (amount, duration)
- High-risk group
- Medication (ACE inhibitor, expectorant)

Examination

- Temperature
- Pulse rate
- Blood pressure in adults (particularly older adults)
- Capillary refill time in children
- Cyanosis (bluish tinge to fingers or lips, indicating poor oxygenation)
- Respiratory rate
- Breathlessness
- Percussion
- Subcostal/intercostal recession (especially in babies)
- Use of accessory muscles
- Crackles or wheezing in chest (and where located)
- Asymmetrical breath sounds/bronchial breathing

Tests

- Peak flow rate if wheezing heard in adult or child over 7 years (see section on asthma exacerbation, later in this chapter)
- Oxygen saturation
- Sputum culture is unhelpful except in special cases (e.g. cystic fibrosis or bronchiectasis, or if tuberculosis is suspected)
- Consider chest x-ray if:
  - Smoker over 50 *or*
  - Cough duration >3 weeks *or*
  - Sputum bloodstained

SPECIFIC TYPES OF COUGH

Cough is a very common problem; other symptoms may accompany it and help to make a diagnosis. The patient may seek help because the cough is persistent, interferes with sleep or because of anxiety that infection is 'going to the chest'. Quite often a friend or a relative has suggested that the patient should seek medical help. Mothers may fear that their children may choke in the night.

Acute cough (less than 3 weeks' duration) may be due to:

- Upper respiratory tract infections, for example, the common cold (viral), which is discussed in Chapter 5
- Acute bronchitis (usually viral)
- Acute laryngitis (viral), associated with hoarseness
- Pneumonia (viral or bacterial)
- Croup in children (viral)
- Bronchiolitis in children (viral)
- Exacerbations of asthma (viral)
- Exacerbations of chronic obstructive pulmonary disease (COPD) or bronchiectasis (bacterial)
- Physical and chemical stimuli, for example, cold air, cigarette smoke
- Pulmonary embolism: unilateral pleuritic chest pain, dry cough, dyspnoea and sometimes haemoptysis
- Remember that the cough of more chronic causes will always seem acute if you see the patient during the first 3 weeks!

A persistent or relapsing cough may occur in:

- Post-viral cough, which may last for several weeks. Patients may expect proprietary cough medicines to cure the cough and come for something stronger because brand X 'hasn't worked'. They need gentle re-education. Cough medicines for chesty coughs (expectorants) can exacerbate cough
- Angiotensin-converting enzyme (ACE) inhibitor therapy (drug names ending in -pril). If the cough goes away immediately after the stopping the drug, then you can be sure it was **not** the drug in the first place (usually takes 1–4 weeks but can take months to resolve)
- Heart failure may cause a persistent cough, with fine crackles at both lung bases and a typical history of being worse when lying down and producing frothy, non-purulent sputum
- Pertussis (whooping cough) – see pertussis section at the end of this chapter
- *Mycoplasma pneumoniae*, an unusual type of infection that occurs in cycles of 3–5 years. It causes a cough that may last for 3 months. It is sensitive to clarithromycin or doxycycline but not amoxicillin. A 2-week course is necessary
- Tuberculosis (TB) – consider this in contacts of people with TB and people born (or who have spent time living) in Asia or Africa. It can be reactivated when immunosuppressed. May be accompanied by weight loss and night sweats
- Asthma (young children may present with cough without wheezing, often worse at night)
- Heavy smokers (but beware cancer and consider COPD)
- Allergic rhinitis (will often have typical 'hay fever' symptoms and seasonal timing if due to pollen)
- Acid reflux may be accompanied by sore throat or heartburn symptoms. However, it can be silent with patient having no indigestion pain or other typical symptoms
- Lung cancer. A persistent cough in a smoker, associated with chest pain, haemoptysis or weight loss, is suspicious
- Habit/tic/oversensitivity of throat

Self-care for coughs

- Most acute coughs are due to the common cold or acute bronchitis; although acute bronchitis may sometimes be caused by bacteria, antibiotics provide little benefit in this condition unless there is co-morbidity
- Adequate fluid intake
- Stop smoking (includes parents of coughing child)
- Soothing drinks, for example, honey and lemon (do not advise honey for child aged under 1 year)
- Some people find linctuses helpful, for example, simple linctus. However, expectorants stimulate sputum production and may contribute to a persistent cough
- Menthol, either inhaled or in a linctus, has a short-lived cough suppressant effect
- Chocolate (contains theobromine) and alcohol may help – maybe liqueur chocolates?
- Pelargonium extract (Kaloba) has been shown in two trials (Timmer et al., 2013) to reduce sputum production in acute bronchitis and there is some evidence to support using andrographis paniculata and ivy/primrose/thyme herbal medicines (Wagner et al., 2015) but they may be difficult to obtain. The interactions of herbal medicines are not well understood, so they are best avoided if other regular medicines (particularly warfarin) are taken
- Remember to give worsening advice – bacterial secondary infection can happen after a viral respiratory tract infection

References

Dicpinigaitis, P. 2006. Angiotensin converting enzyme inhibitor-induced cough: ACCP evidence-based clinical practice guidelines. *Chest*; 129(1 Suppl): 169S–173S. http://journal.chestnet.org/article/S0012-3692(15)52845-6/fulltext. doi: 10.1378/chest.129.1_suppl.169S.

Morice, A. 2016. It's time to change the way we approach coughs in community pharmacy. *Pharm J*. www.pharmaceutical-journal.com/opinion/insight/its-time-to-change-the-way-we-approach-coughs-in-community-pharmacy/20200821.article.

Oduwole, O., Udoh, E.E., Oyo-Ita, A., and Meremikwu, M.M. 2018. Honey for acute cough in children. *Cochrane Database Syst Rev*; 4. Art. No.: CD007094. DOI: 10.1002/14651858.CD007094.pub5.

Robertson, S., Robinson, M., Schultz, A., and Villella, R. 2016. Do over-the-counter remedies relieve cough in acute upper respiratory infections? *Evid Based Pract*; 19(9). https://mospace.umsystem.edu/xmlui/bitstream/handle/10355/59387/EBP-September-2016-01.pdf?sequence=1.

Timmer, A., Günther, J., Motschall, E., Rücker, G., Antes, G., and Kern, W. 2013. Pelargonium sidoides extract for treating acute respiratory tract infections. *Cochrane Database Syst Rev*; (10): Art. No.: CD006323. doi: 10.1002/14651858.CD006323.pub3.

Wagner, L., Cramer, H., Klose, P., Lauche, R., Gass, F., Dobos, G., and Langhorst, J. 2015. Herbal medicine for cough: A systematic review and meta-analysis. *Complementary Medicine Research*; 22(6):359–68.

ACUTE BRONCHITIS

- A viral or bacterial infection of adults or children
- Fever
- Cough (may be productive)
- Maybe wheeze
- Maybe central chest pain on coughing
- No other chest signs
- Normal respiratory rate, pulse and blood pressure (BP)
- The commonest diagnosis in acute cough (Figure 4.1). An antibiotic is not usually indicated (Box 4.1)

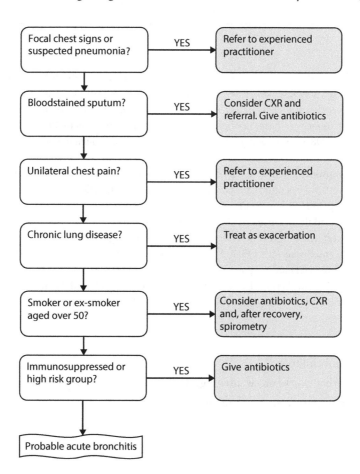

Figure 4.1 Adult with acute cough – is it acute bronchitis?

BOX 4.1 ANTIBIOTICS FOR ACUTE BRONCHITIS

Prescribe an antibiotic if:

- Seriously ill
- High-risk group (see Chapter 2)
- Bloodstained sputum

Consider an antibiotic if:

- Smoker aged over 50 (may have undiagnosed COPD – consider chest x-ray (CXR) now and then spirometry 6 weeks after recovery from acute infection)
- Prolonged (>3 weeks) or worsening symptoms

Antibiotic choice

- Amoxicillin for 5 days (500 mg three times daily for adults). See Members' section of NMIC website for debate about doxycycline
- If allergic to penicillin, then use clarithromycin[PIQ] (250 mg twice daily for adults) or doxycycline[PBC] (200 mg on the first day then 100 mg once daily)
- If not responding to amoxicillin, add clarithromycin[PIQ]

 RED FLAGS

- Persistent symptoms (*consider whooping cough, tuberculosis and lung cancer*)
- Weight loss (*consider tuberculosis, lung cancer and autoimmune disease*)
- Unexplained haemoptysis (*consider 2-week wait lung cancer referral*)
- Previous asbestos exposure (*CXR for lung cancer and mesothelioma*)

References

Cornford, C.S., Morgan, M., and Ridsdale, L. 1993. Why do mothers consult when their children cough? *Fam Pract*; 10(2): 193–196. http://europepmc.org/abstract/MED/8359610?europe_pmc_extredirect=https://doi.org/10.1093/fampra/10.2.193. doi: 10.1093/fampra/10.2.193. *An old paper (but still the best) which gives fascinating insights into parents' concerns.*

Johnson, G., and Helman, C. 2004. Remedy or cure? Lay beliefs about over-the-counter medicines for coughs and colds. *BJGP*; 54: 98–102. http://bjgp.org/content/54/499/98. *Common confusion between the ability of a medicine to relieve symptoms, and its ability to cure a disease or to hasten recovery.*

Little, P., Stuart, B., Smith, S., Thompson, M., Knox, K., van den Bruel, A., Lown, M., Moore, M., and Mant, D. 2017. Antibiotic prescription strategies and adverse outcome for uncomplicated lower respiratory tract infections: Prospective cough complication cohort (3C) study. *BMJ*; 357: j2148. doi.org/10.1136/bmj.j2148.

NICE CKS. 2015. Chest infections – adult. cks.nice.org.uk/chest-infections-adult.

NICE NG12. 2017. Suspected cancer: Recognition and referral. www.nice.org.uk/guidance/ng12.

Smith, S.M., Fahey, T., Smucny, J., and Becker, L.A. 2017. Antibiotics for acute bronchitis. *Cochrane Database Syst Rev*; Issue 6. Art. No.: CD000245. doi: 10.1002/14651858.CD000245.pub4.

Usmani, O., Belvisi, M., Patel, H., Crispino, N., Birrell, M., Korbonits, M., Korbonits, D., and Barnes, P. 2005. Theobromine inhibits sensory nerve activation and cough. *FASEB J*; 19: 231–233. doi: 10.1096/fj.04-1990fje.

LARYNGITIS

- A viral infection of adults and children
- History: hoarseness, sore throat (worse on swallowing), fever, headache and dry irritating cough
- Examination: usually normal apart from fever and hoarse voice
- Self-care:
  - Rest voice
  - Avoid smoky environments
  - Drink adequate fluids

- Try not to swallow or cough more than essential
- Take paracetamol or ibuprofen[P] if needed for headache or throat pain

RED FLAGS

- Aged 45 and over with persistent unexplained hoarseness (*2-week wait head and neck cancer referral*)
- Actual difficulty swallowing (not related to pain). This may be worse for solids than liquids (*2-week wait upper GI cancer referral*)

References

NICE NG12. 2017. Suspected cancer: Recognition and referral. www.nice.org.uk/guidance/ng12.

Reveiz, L., and Cardona, A. 2015. Antibiotics for acute laryngitis in adults. *Cochrane Database Syst Rev*; (5): Art. No.: CD004783. doi: 10.1002/14651858.CD004783.pub5.

PNEUMONIA

- An infection of the lung parenchyma, usually bacterial
- High mortality
- History: fever, rigors, cough, breathlessness, bloodstained or rusty sputum, unilateral chest pain, muscle or joint pain
- Examination: fever, rapid respiration, tachycardia and focal chest signs (e.g., dullness on percussion, bronchial breathing, coarse crackles)
- Elderly people may have non-specific symptoms and are less likely to have fever
- CRB-65 score for mortality risk (Table 4.1) – one point for each of:
  - Confusion (new disorientation)
  - Raised respiratory rate ($\geq$30/min)
  - Low blood pressure (diastolic $\leq$60 mmHg or systolic <90 mmHg)
  - Age $\geq$65 years
  - Consider admission if score $\geq$1, especially if $\geq$2

Table 4.1 Predictive value of CRB-65 score on mortality from pneumonia in hospital patients

CRB-65 score	Risk of mortality (%)	Antibiotic choice
0	1	Single
1	5	Dual
2	12	Dual
3	18	Dual
4	33	Dual

Tests

- Oxygen saturation
- Consider C-reactive protein (CRP) blood test if it is available and there is diagnostic uncertainty (Table 4.2)
- If smoker aged over 50, arrange chest x-ray now and then spirometry appointment when recovered
- If pneumonia is confirmed, a repeat chest x-ray is advised after 6 weeks

Table 4.2 Interpreting CRP blood test results in people with symptoms of lower respiratory tract infection

CRP result (mg/L)	Risk of mortality (%)	Action
<20	<1	No antibiotic
20–100	1	Offer delayed antibiotic
>100	10–19	Offer antibiotic and consider admission

Self-care

- Maintain adequate fluid intake
- Avoid physical exertion until the fever settles
- Advise on the likely progress:
  - 1 week – fever should have resolved
  - 4 weeks – chest pain and sputum production should have substantially reduced
  - 3 months – most symptoms should have resolved, but fatigue might still be present
  - 6 months – symptoms should have fully resolved

Action

- Offer an antibiotic, unless this is inappropriate (e.g. comfort care on an end-of-life pathway)
- Review within 3 days
- Advise the patient to seek medical advice within 3 days if symptoms do not begin to improve, or earlier if symptoms worsen as hospital admission may be needed

Antibiotic choice

- Amoxicillin for 5–7 days (500 mg – 1 g three times daily for adults)
- If allergic to penicillin, then use clarithromycin[PIQ] (500 mg twice daily for adults)
- If not responding to amoxicillin, add clarithromycin[PIQ]
- In more severe pneumonia, amoxicillin plus clarithromycin[PIQ] for 7–10 days. If allergic to penicillin, then use doxycycline[PBC] for seven days (200 mg on the first day then 100 mg once daily)
- If following flu-like illness, use co-amoxiclav (500/125 mg three times daily for adults), not amoxicillin, which does not cover *Staphylococcus*. If patient is allergic to penicillin, then use doxycycline[PBC] for adults or clarithromycin[PIQ] for children
- Review treatment at 7 days and consider extending to 14–21 days

RED FLAGS

- Severe illness, breathlessness or confusion (*severe illness; admit Medical or Paediatrics*)
- Worsening despite oral treatment (*needs intravenous (IV) antibiotic; admit Medical or Paediatrics*)
- Patient with HIV (*possible Pneumocystis jiroveci pneumonia; admit Medical or Paediatrics*)
- Unilateral chest pain, worse on coughing or deep breathing (*suggests pleurisy; pulmonary embolism; or pneumothorax; consider hospital assessment*)
- Recession (*unusual; suggests alternative diagnosis; for example, bronchiolitis*)
- Signs of sepsis (see Chapter 3) (*admit*)
- Oxygen saturation below 94% (*admit*)
- CRB-65 score ≥1 (*consider admission; especially if ≥2*)
- CRP result >100 (*consider admission; especially if very high*)
- Baby with abnormal chest examination (*differential diagnosis includes bronchiolitis; refer to senior colleague*)

Caution

Pneumonia is not a minor illness and should only be managed by experienced clinicians.

References

Blackburn, R., Henderson, K., Lillie, M., Sheridan, E., George, R., Deas, A., and Johnson, A. 2011. Empirical treatment of influenza-associated pneumonia in primary care: A descriptive study of the antimicrobial susceptibility of lower respiratory tract bacteria (England, Wales and Northern Ireland, January 2007–March 2010). *Thorax*; 66: 389–395. http://thorax.bmj.com/content/66/5/389. doi: 10.1136/thx.2010.134643.

Chalmers, J., Singanayam, A., and Hill, A. 2008. C-reactive protein is an independent predictor of severity in community-acquired pneumonia. *Am J Med*; 121: 219–225. http://infekt.ch/content/uploads/2013/11/jc_mai09_schweizer.pdf. doi: 10.1016/j.amjmed.2007.10.033.

NICE CG191. 2014. Pneumonia in adults: Diagnosis and management. www.nice.org.uk/guidance/cg191.

NICE CKS. 2017. Chest infections – adult and cough – acute with chest signs in children.

COPD/BRONCHIECTASIS EXACERBATION

History
- Sputum quantity, colour and thickness
- Breathlessness
- Fever
- Recent antibiotics/have they taken their rescue antibiotics?
- Previous episodes and their treatment
- Care plan in place?

Examination
- Temperature
- Confusion
- Cyanosis
- Ankle oedema
- Respiratory rate/distress
- Wheezing
- Pursed lip breathing
- Use of accessory muscles
- Oxygen saturation (compare with their usual)

Test
- Sputum culture is helpful before starting an antibiotic (especially if the infection turns out to respond poorly to initial treatment), and should always be sent for exacerbations of bronchiectasis

Self-care
- Increase dose or frequency of short-acting bronchodilator to the maximum (salbutamol or ipratropium)
- Use a spacer
- Worsening advice

Prescription
- If breathlessness has worsened, give prednisolone[I] 30 mg/day for 7–14 days

***

 BOX 4.2 ANTIBIOTICS FOR COPD/BRONCHIECTASIS EXACERBATIONS

Prescribe an antibiotic:

- If sputum has become purulent (green and thick)

***

Antibiotic choice
Be guided by the result of the most recent sputum culture, or if none, then what treatment proved helpful in the previous infective episode.

- Amoxicillin for 5 days (500 mg three times daily for adults)
- If allergic to penicillin, use doxycycline[PBC] (200 mg on the first day then 100 mg once daily) or clarithromycin[PIQ] (500 mg twice daily for adults)
- If severe COPD with recurrent antibiotic use, consider co-amoxiclav (500/125 mg three times daily for adults)
- If not responding to amoxicillin, add clarithromycin[PIQ] or change to doxycycline[PBC]

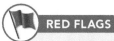

RED FLAGS

- New confusion (*admit under Medical or Paediatrics*)
- Severe symptoms/increasing oedema/significant comorbidity/living alone (*consider admission*)
- Cyanosis, or oxygen saturation <95% (depending on their usual reading and your confidence in managing these patients) (*consider cautious oxygen and hospital admission if saturation <90%*)

References

NICE CG101. 2010. Chronic obstructive pulmonary disease in over 16s: Diagnosis and management. www.nice.org.uk/guidance/cg101.

Wedzicha, J., Miravitlles, M., Hurst, J., Calverley, P., Albert, R., Anzueto, A., Criner, G. et al. 2017. Management of COPD exacerbations: A European Respiratory Society/American Thoracic Society guideline. *Eur Respir J*; 49(3). http://erj.ersjournals.com/lens/erj/49/3/1600791. doi: 10.1183/13993003.00791-2016. *Support for the use of oral corticosteroids and antibiotics for exacerbations.*

ASTHMA EXACERBATION

History

- Cough
- Wheeze
- Breathlessness
- Sleep disturbance
- Fever
- Previous hospital admissions for asthma
- Any previous intensive care admissions
- Current medication
- Asthma action plan?

Examination

- Agitation
- Ability to complete sentence
- Cyanosis
- Respiratory rate
- Recession/use of accessory muscles
- Pulse rate and blood pressure in severe episodes
- Peak flow
- Oxygen saturation

Self-care

- Immediately use salbutamol inhaler with a spacer if available:
  - One puff at a time and inhale with five tidal breaths via spacer
  - Adult: 4 puffs initially, followed by two puffs every 2 minutes according to response, up to 10 puffs, each delivered individually if using spacer

    Child: 2 puffs every 2 minutes according to response, up to 10 puffs
  - Repeat every 10–20 minutes according to response
- Afterwards:
  - Use inhaled salbutamol as required, up to four times a day (not more frequently than every four hours)
  - Do not increase the dose of inhaled steroid – this is ineffective acutely and oral steroids are preferable here
  - Worsening advice: monitor peak expiratory flow rate (PEFR) and symptoms. If symptoms worsen or PEFR decreases, seek further advice

Prescription

- Do not give antibiotics unless there are signs of pneumonia
- Do not alter the dose of inhaled corticosteroid acutely; continue the patient's usual inhaled dose while on oral steroids
- Give a short course of oral prednisolone[1]:
  - Child <2 years: 10 mg daily for 3 days
  - Child 2–5 years: 20 mg daily for 3 days
  - Child 6–12 years: 30–40 mg daily for 3 days
  - Adult or child >12 years: 40–50 mg daily for 5 days

Arrange follow-up within 48 hours. Once recovered, will need further review (after about a month) to adjust medication and potentially update asthma action plan.

RED FLAGS

Consider nebulized salbutamol driven with oxygen and transfer to hospital if:

- Peak flow less than 50% of best or predicted
- Exhaustion, using accessory muscles, or inability to complete a sentence
- Brittle asthma with previous hospital admission (*particularly intensive care*)
- Living alone/social issues
- Oxygen saturation <95% or cyanosis
- Pregnancy
- No response to bronchodilator

Reference

British Thoracic Society (BTS) and Scottish Intercollegiate Guidelines Network (SIGN). 2016. British guideline on the management of asthma. www.brit-thoracic.org.uk/standards-of-care/guidelines/btssign-british-guideline-on-the-management-of-asthma.

VIRAL-INDUCED WHEEZE

Viral infections may cause wheezing and tightness in the chest in those who do not have asthma. Use salbutamol metered-dose inhaler (MDI) via spacer, four times daily for one week. Consider montelukast in those who cannot accept an inhaler. In children, those with a family history of atopy and exercise-induced wheeze are more likely to develop asthma later.

DIFFERENTIAL DIAGNOSIS OF ACUTE COUGH IN CHILDREN

As well as the conditions mentioned previously, there are certain illnesses that may cause acute cough in children: bronchiolitis, croup and whooping cough (Table 4.3).

Table 4.3 Differential diagnosis of acute cough with chest signs in children

	Pneumonia	Bronchiolitis	Viral-induced wheeze
Age	Any age	Under 1 year	12 months–5 years
Fever	Yes	Yes	Maybe
Respiratory rate	Increased	Increased	Normal or increased
Recession	No	Maybe	Maybe
Hyperinflation	No	Often	Maybe
Wheeze	No[a]	Maybe	Present
Crackles	Coarse, localised	Fine, generalised	None

[a] Except with Mycoplasma pneumoniae.

BRONCHIOLITIS

- A viral infection of children under 2 years, mainly 3–6 months
- Mainly caused by respiratory syncytial virus

History

- Persistent cough following an upper respiratory tract infection (URTI)
- May be breathless or have episodes of apnoea

Examination

- Temperature
- Capillary refill time
- Respiratory rate
- Recession/use of accessory muscles
- Chest – often scattered crackles and wheezes
- Percussion – no dullness
- Oxygen saturation (controversial – see Quinonez et al., 2017)

Self-care

- Maintain adequate fluid intake
- There is no specific treatment. Steam inhalations are no longer recommended (Al Himdani et al., 2016)
- This is a long illness: only 50% of children will be better by day 13
- Worsening advice, to look for:
    - Faster breathing (specific advice follows)
    - Increasing difficulty in breathing
    - Recession
    - Reduced feeding (less than 50% of normal)
    - Signs of dehydration
    - Worsening fever

RED FLAGS

- Fever >39°C or focal signs in chest (*possible pneumonia; refer to senior clinician*)
- Apnoea (*admit*)
- Recession or tachypnoea: 0–5 months >60/min, 6–12 months >50/min, >12 months >40/min (*consider admission*)
- Oxygen saturation <92% (*give oxygen and admit*)

References

Al Himdani, S., Javed, M., Hughes, J., Falconer, O., Bidder, C., Hemington-Gorse, S., and Nguyen, D. 2016. Home remedy or hazard? Management and costs of paediatric steam inhalation therapy burn injuries. *Br J Gen Pract*; 66(644): e193–e199. http://bjgp.org/content/66/644/e193.long. doi: 10.3399/bjgp16X684289.

CKS. 2017. Cough (acute) with chest signs in children. cks.nice.org.uk/cough-acute-with-chest-signs-in-children

NICE NG9. 2015. Bronchiolitis in children: Diagnosis and management. www.nice.org.uk/guidance/ng9.

Quinonez, R., Coon, E., Schroeder, A., and Moyer, V. 2017. When technology creates uncertainty: Pulse oximetry and overdiagnosis of hypoxaemia in bronchiolitis. *BMJ*; 358: j3850. doi.org/10.1136/bmj.j3850.

Thompson, M., Vodicka Talley, A., Blair, P.S., Buckley David, I., Carl, H., Hay, A.D. et al. 2013. Duration of symptoms of respiratory tract infections in children: Systematic review. *BMJ*; 347: f7027. doi.org/10.1136/bmj.f7027.

Umoren, R., Odey, F., and Meremikwu, M. 2011. Steam inhalation or humidified oxygen for acute bronchiolitis in children up to three years of age. *Cochrane Database Syst Rev*; (1): Art. No.: CD006435.

CROUP

A viral infection of children aged between 3 months and 5 years.

History
- Cough (often brassy or barking)
- Crowing noise on inspiration (stridor, worse at night)
- Fever
- May be breathless

Examination
- Temperature
- Capillary refill time
- Respiratory rate
- Recession/use of accessory muscles
- Chest (usually normal)
- Oxygen saturation
- Throat

Self-care
- Explain nature of illness
- Steam inhalations are no longer recommended
- Worsening advice

Prescription
- Give all children with croup a single dose of oral dexamethasone[I] (150 micrograms/kg). Tablets are available as 500 micrograms and 2 mg. Round the dose up to the nearest tablet available. We would caution against prescribing soluble tablets or liquid preparations because pharmacies may not stock them, and ordinary tablets dissolve in water adequately for young children
- If dexamethasone is unavailable, give two doses of oral prednisolone[I] (1–2 mg/kg) 24 hours apart

RED FLAGS

Consider admission to hospital if:

- Abnormal airway (*including Down's syndrome*)
- Distress/agitation
- Immunosuppressed
- Severe recession
- Respiratory distress
- Parents not coping

References

Garbutt, J.M., Conlon, B., Sterkel, R., Baty, J., Schechtman, K.B., Mandrell, K., Leege, E., Gentry, S., and Stunk, R.C. 2013. The comparative effectiveness of prednisolone and dexamethasone for children with croup: a community-based randomized trial. *Clin Paediatr*; 52(11), 1014–1021.

Moore, M., and Little, P. 2007. Humidified air inhalation for treating croup: A systematic review and meta-analysis. *Fam Pract*; 24(4): 295–301. https://academic.oup.com/fampra/article-lookup/doi/10.1093/fampra/cmm022.

NICE CKS. 2012. Croup. https://cks.nice.org.uk/croup.

Russell, K., Liang, Y., O'Gorman, K., Johnson, D., and Klassen, T. 2011. Glucocorticoids for croup. *Cochrane Database Syst Rev*; (1): Art. No.: CD001955. doi: 10.1002/14651858.CD001955.pub3.

WHOOPING COUGH

A bacterial infection caused by *Bordetella pertussis* affecting all ages, most commonly babies under 3 months old who are too young to be directly protected by routine immunization.

- Underdiagnosed
- Consider in child if coughing >2 weeks, especially if sputum is thick and vomiting occurs after coughing
- Median duration of cough: 112 days
- Examination of chest is usually normal
- Notifiable disease

Tests

- Public Health England guidance (2018) states that pertussis serology will no longer be available at NHS expense. A new oral fluid test is available; the choice of test has become very complex. See appendix 6 of PHE (2018)

Self-care

- Stay away from day care, school or work for 2 days after starting antibiotics, or 21 days after the onset of cough, whichever is the sooner
- Expect recovery to take several weeks

Prescription

- Clarithromycin[PIQ] for 7 days (500 mg twice daily for adults): if given in the first 3 weeks of illness, it reduces transmission but does not benefit the patient

References

Harnden, A., Grant, C., Harrison, T., Brueggemann, A., Mayon-White, R., and Mant, D. 2006. Whooping cough in school age children with persistent cough: Prospective cohort study in primary care. *BMJ*; 300: 174–177. www.bmj.com/content/333/7560/174. doi: 10.1136/bmj.38870.655405.AE.

Public Health England. 2016. Pertussis factsheet for healthcare professionals. www.gov.uk/government/uploads/system/uploads/attachment_data/file/562472/HCW_Factsheet_Pertussis.pdf.

Public Health England. 2018. Guidance for the public health management of pertussis in England. https://assets.publishing.service.gov.uk/government/uploads/system/uploads/attachment_data/file/704482/Guidelines_for_the_public_health_management_of_pertussis_in_England.pdf.

CHAPTER 5

Ear, nose and throat

SORE THROAT

History

- Patient's agenda – often pain relief
- Duration
- Fever
- Rash
- Medication already tried
- Other symptoms such as cough or blocked/discharging nose
- ⚑ Drooling/unable to swallow
- ⚑ Structural heart disease: previous heart valve problems/endocarditis/cardiomyopathy
- ⚑ Immunosuppressed
- ⚑ Medication that may affect the bone marrow (agranulocytosis), for example, immunosuppressants (including corticosteroids), carbimazole, mirtazapine, sulfasalazine, clozapine and disease-modifying antirheumatic drugs (DMARDs)

Examination

- Temperature (consider any recent antipyretic)
- Examine throat – asking the patient to yawn, take a deep breath or pant may improve the view. Consider using a tongue depressor on the sides of the tongue if back of throat not visible (but exclude epiglottitis first, see below). Assess inflammation of pharynx and look for exudates on tonsils
- Check neck for enlarged lymph nodes (cervical lymphadenopathy)
- Look for the rash of scarlet fever (small rough pinpricks)

Test

- Urgent full blood count (FBC) should be requested if taking medication potentially toxic to bone marrow. The safest course of action is usually to stop the potentially toxic drug until the FBC result is confirmed to be normal
- Rapid antigen throat swab tests designed to detect Streptococcus are unreliable and should not be used

Self-care advice

- Most sore throats are viral. Symptoms resolve within 3 days in 40% of people and within 7 days in 85%, irrespective of whether the sore throat is viral or due to a streptococcal infection
- Ibuprofen[P] or paracetamol can relieve pain
- Warm saltwater mouthwash (half a teaspoon of salt in 250 ml water)
- Cold drinks and ice lollies may be soothing
- Benzydamine mouthwash or spray (e.g. Difflam® OTC) may relieve the discomfort
- Flurbiprofen[PBC] lozenges (Strefen® OTC) are an alternative (one 8.75 mg lozenge every 3–6 hours for maximum 3 days, allow lozenge to dissolve slowly in the mouth; maximum five lozenges per day). Adverse events occurred in around 40% of people using flurbiprofen lozenges, including taste disturbances, numbness, dry mouth and nausea (NICE, 2018)
- Oral corticosteroids may be prescribed if the pain is very severe but carry significant risks of sepsis and venous thromboembolism
- Worsening advice: seek help if they develop difficulty in breathing or are unable to swallow enough fluid to maintain hydration

Bacterial or viral infection?

Antibiotics are generally of marginal benefit in sore throat and may only shorten the illness by 16 hours (remember that the immune system is designed to handle sore throats, both viral and bacterial in origin, and is usually highly competent in doing so). Against this must be weighed the cost to the patient (prescription charge, burden of medicine-taking, risk of side effects) and to society (antibiotic resistance, medicalisation of self-limiting illness). Viral infection is the commonest cause of sore throat (75% of children and 90% of adults). Clinical scores and point-of-care tests have been developed with the aim of identifying those patients more likely to benefit from antibiotics. Harmless, commensal streptococci are present in the throats of 12%–40% of healthy people. Rapid antigen tests for *group A streptococcus* are not recommended by national guidance because they are unable to distinguish between pathogens and commensals, and they do not detect types of streptococci other than group A. Thus, throat swabs are not usually helpful.

NICE (2018) recommends the use of either Centor criteria or the FeverPAIN score (Box 5.1) to guide the management of sore throat. Public Health England (2017) favours the FeverPAIN score.

BOX 5.1 FeverPAIN SCORE (Little et al., 2013)

One point for each of:

- Fever in last 24 hours
- Purulence
- Attends with symptoms rapidly (under 3 days)
- Inflammation of tonsils (if severe)
- No cough or coryza

Score of 0–1: only 13%–18% have Streptococcus (close to background carriage); no antibiotic.
Score of 2–3: 34%–40% have Streptococcus; consider delayed antibiotic.
Score of >4: 62%–65% have Streptococcus; consider immediate antibiotic if severe symptoms or delayed antibiotic prescription.

Action: See Box 5.2

 BOX 5.2 ANTIBIOTICS FOR SORE THROAT

Prescribe an antibiotic if:

- Seriously ill
- Prolonged and worsening symptoms
- Immunosuppressed
- Structural heart disease: *risk of endocarditis*

Consider an antibiotic if:

- FeverPAIN score 4 or more

Antibiotic choice

- Phenoxymethylpenicillin (penicillin V) for 5–10 days (500 mg four times daily for adults) (see members' section of NMIC website for debate on duration)
- If allergic to penicillin, use clarithromycin[PIQ] for 5 days (250 mg twice daily for adults)
- For children who are unable to swallow tablets, amoxicillin suspension may be used instead. It tastes much better than phenoxymethylpenicillin suspension, and concordance is likely to be better because it is given three times daily. Avoid if glandular fever is suspected (see section on Other Types of Sore Throat below)
- If not responding to antibiotic, reassess. Viral causes are common and are the usual reason for poor response. If a second antibiotic is thought necessary from the degree of inflammation and systemic symptoms and signs, use metronidazole[Q] for 7 days (400 mg three times daily for adults)

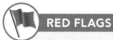
RED FLAGS

- Drooling, cannot swallow, respiratory distress (*possible epiglottitis; do not examine throat; call 999*)
- Large swelling around one tonsil, feverish and unwell (*possible quinsy; refer same day to ear, nose and throat [ENT] team*)
- Structural heart disease (*risk of endocarditis; prescribe antibiotic and discuss with senior colleague*)
- Taking medication that may be toxic to bone marrow (*urgent full blood count [FBC]; seek urgent advice*)

References

Aertgeerts, B., Agoritsas, T., Siemieniuk, R., Burgers, J., Bekkering, G., Merglen, A., van Driel, M. et al. 2017. Corticosteroids for sore throat: A clinical practice guideline *BMJ*; 358:j4090. doi.org/10.1136/bmj.j4090. *This controversial guideline recommends giving high-dose dexamethasone to reduce the symptoms of sore throat. However, in NMIC's opinion, the possible benefits do not outweigh the risks.*

Lan, A.J., Colford, J.M., Colford, J.M. Jr. 2000. The impact of dosing frequency on the efficacy of 10-day penicillin or amoxicillin therapy for streptococcal tonsillopharyngitis: A meta-analysis. *Pediatrics*; 105(2):E19. *This meta-analysis provides some evidence that twice daily dosing with phenoxymethylpenicillin is at least as effective as four times daily in treating GABHS. However, Public Health England has recommended that four times daily dosage is used.*

Little, P., Hobbs, R., Moore, M., Mant, D., Williamson, I., McNulty, C., Cheng, Y.E. et al. 2013. Clinical score and rapid antigen detection test to guide antibiotic use for sore throats: Randomised controlled trial of PRISM (primary care streptococcal management). *BMJ*; 347:f5806. doi.org/10.1136/bmj.f5806. *Evidence for the Fever/PAIN score. Lack of evidence for the rapid antigen test.*

NICE CG64. 2017. Prophylaxis against infective endocarditis: Antimicrobial prophylaxis against infective endocarditis in adults and children undergoing interventional procedures. www.nice.org.uk/guidance/cg64. *This guidance states that any episodes of infection in people at risk of infective endocarditis should be treated promptly to reduce the risk of endocarditis developing.*

NICE NG84. 2018. Sore throat (acute): Antimicrobial prescribing. www.nice.org.uk/guidance/ng84.

Public Health England. 2017. Management of infection guidance for primary care for consultation and local adaptation. www.gov.uk/government/uploads/system/uploads/attachment_data/file/612743/Managing_common_infections.pdf.

Roggen, I., van Berlaer, G., Gordts, F., Pierard, D., and Hubloue, L. 2013. Centor criteria in children in a paediatric emergency department: For what it is worth. *BMJ Open*; 3:e002712. doi: 10.1136/bmjopen-2013-002712. *The Centor score was of no value in identifying children with bacterial sore throats.*

Shephard, A., Smith, G., Aspley, S., and Schachtel, B.P. 2015. Randomised, double-blind, placebo-controlled studies on flurbiprofen 8.75 mg lozenges in patients with/without group A or C streptococcal throat infection, with an assessment of clinicians' prediction of 'strep throat'. *Int J Clin Pract*; 69:59–71. doi: 10.1111/ijcp.12536. *A single flurbiprofen lozenge provided better pain relief than placebo.*

Spinks, A., Glasziou, P.P., and Del Mar, C.B. 2013. Antibiotics for sore throat. *Cochrane Database Syst Rev*; (11). Art. No.: CD000023. doi: 10.1002/14651858.CD000023.pub4.

OTHER TYPES OF SORE THROAT

1. Glandular fever
2. Quinsy
3. Epiglottitis

GLANDULAR FEVER

- Age 15–25 most commonly affected
- Often asymptomatic
- Caused by Epstein-Barr virus
- Long incubation period (1–2 months)
- Transmission by saliva

History

- Fever
- Neck pain due to enlarged lymph nodes
- Sore throat
- Malaise and fatigue

Examination

- Enlarged tonsils with exudate
- Generalised lymphadenopathy, especially posterior neck nodes
- Oedema of the uvula or around the eyes
- Petechial rash on the palate
- Variable generalised skin rash
- Jaundice may be visible

Tests

- Full blood count (glandular fever is likely if 20% of lymphocytes are atypical or reactive)
- Paul Bunnell or Monospot blood test, after at least 7 days (slow to turn positive and high false-negative rate)
- Epstein-Barr virus serology (useful where the previous tests leave the diagnosis in doubt and there is need to identify the virus, for example, in pregnancy). (Glandular fever is not harmful in pregnancy, but cytomegalovirus may cause similar symptoms)

Cautions

- Risk of rupture of spleen or respiratory obstruction from large tonsils
- Avoid strenuous activity and contact sports (e.g. rugby) for 4 weeks
- Avoid spread of infection from saliva
- Avoid amoxicillin and ampicillin, which may cause a rash (the rash is disease-specific, not due to an allergy)

References

Lennon, P., Crotty, M., and Fenton, J.E. 2015. Infectious mononucleosis. *BMJ*; 350:h1825. doi: 10.1136/bmj.h1825.
Public Health England UK. 2015. Standards for microbiology investigations: Epstein-Barr virus serology. *Virology*; 26(5):1–13. *Useful flow chart and table to help interpretation of test results.*

QUINSY (PERITONSILLAR ABSCESS)

- History of unilateral sore throat (usually)
- Severe illness with high fever
- 'Hot potato' voice and offensive breath
- Trismus (unable to open mouth)
- May have earache on the affected side
- Deviated uvula
- ⚑ Refer same day to ENT

EPIGLOTTITIS

- Rarely seen in children now (due to Hib vaccination), more often in adults
- Check vaccination history, especially if not exposed to UK childhood vaccination schedule
- High fever
- Severe sore throat
- Difficulty and pain when swallowing, maybe drooling
- Tachycardia
- Anterior neck tenderness
- 'Hot potato' voice
- Respiratory distress or stridor
- ⚑ Do not examine the throat
- ⚑ Refer as emergency to ENT and convey via blue light ambulance

MOUTH PROBLEMS

1. Oral candidiasis
2. Aphthous ulcers
3. Herpes simplex stomatitis

Hand, foot and mouth disease – see Chapter 8

ORAL CANDIDIASIS (THRUSH)

A fungal infection common in babies, or anyone using inhaled corticosteroids or oral antibiotics, or who is immunosuppressed.

History
- Soreness in mouth and tongue
- Difficulty in eating/drinking
- Immunosuppressed
- Use of a steroid inhaler for asthma or COPD

Examination
- White patches on tongue and oral mucosa that cannot easily be removed
- Redness of tongue or denture contact areas

Tests
- Swabs are unhelpful because candida is a common commensal
- In adults consider FBC, fasting plasma glucose (FPG) or HbA1c, and human immunodeficiency virus (HIV) serology

Self-care
- Avoid reinfection from teats/nipples/dummies in babies
- Good dental/denture hygiene in adults
- For those using inhaled steroids, recommend spacer (e.g., AeroChamber®) is used and afterwards rinse mouth out with water
- Miconazole[I] oral gel (OTC over age of 4 months) is the most effective treatment. Recommend use for at least 7 days, extending to 14 days if recovery is slow. Continue treatment for at least 2 days after symptoms have resolved

Prescription
- Miconazole[I] oral gel is recommended as first line for all patients (unless taking warfarin, as there is an interaction). In babies, parents should be advised to take care that the gel does not obstruct the throat; avoid application to the back of the throat and subdivide doses. A prescription will be required for babies under 4 months (*unlicensed indication*)
- Nystatin suspension is an alternative but is 50% less effective and not licensed under 1 month
- Oral fluconazole[PIQ] 50–100 mg daily for 7 days may be used in severe or resistant cases in adults

 RED FLAG

- Oral candidiasis is unusual in a healthy adult. Unless there is an obvious trigger, for example, inhaled corticosteroids or recent broad-spectrum antibiotic, offer screening for immunosuppression including HIV

References

Ainsworth, S., and Jones, W. 2009. It sticks in our throats too. *BMJ*; 338:a3178. *Explains why the licence for miconazole was revoked for babies under 4 months.*

Hoppe, J.E. 1997. Treatment of oropharyngeal candidiasis in immunocompetent infants: A randomized multicenter study of miconazole gel vs. nystatin suspension. The Antifungals Study Group. *Pediatr Infect Dis J*; 16(3):288–293. *Miconazole gel was significantly superior to nystatin.*

NICE CKS. 2013. Candida – oral. cks.nice.org.uk/candida-oral.

APHTHOUS ULCERS

History

- Painful mouth ulcers, often recurring since childhood
- About half of those with recurrent ulcers may have a first-degree relative with similar symptoms
- May occur anywhere in the mouth, most commonly on the buccal mucosa (lining of the cheek)
- 🚩 Consider other diagnoses if present >3 weeks or ulcers elsewhere

Examination

- Red, round lesions, sometimes with white crater

Self-care

- Reduce oral trauma (e.g. softer toothbrush)
- If recurrent, notice if any foodstuffs trigger outbreaks, for example, coffee, chocolate, peanuts
- Benzydamine spray (e.g. Difflam® OTC) to reduce pain (for adults four to eight sprays on to affected area every 1.5 to 3 hours)
- Topical anaesthetic gels (e.g. Bonjela^C adult gel® OTC) for adults (apply half an inch with gentle massage, nor more often than every 3 hours). Do not use for children due to risk of Reye's syndrome
- Alternatives that do not contain salicylates (e.g. Bonjela junior gel® OTC) can be safely used for children (apply half an inch with gentle massage, not more often than every 3 hours)
- Chlorhexidine mouthwash (OTC) to prevent secondary bacterial infection. Rinse or gargle 10 ml twice daily (rinse or gargle for about 1 minute)

Prescription

- Hydrocortisone^P mucoadhesive buccal tablets, used at the first sign (one 2.5 mg tablet four times a day, allowed to dissolve slowly in the mouth in contact with the ulcer)

RED FLAGS

- Persisting more than 3 weeks (*2-week wait cancer referral to Oral Surgeon*)
- Ulceration affects other parts of body (*consider alternative diagnoses, for example, coeliac disease, Behçet's disease, reactive arthritis; refer to senior colleague*)

References

NICE CKS. 2012. Aphthous ulcer. cks.nice.org.uk/aphthous-ulcer.

Wardhana, D.E.A. 2010. Recurrent aphthous stomatitis caused by food allergy. *Acta Medica Indonesia*; 42(4):236–240.

HERPES SIMPLEX STOMATITIS

As well as the familiar cold sore (see section on Localised Rashes, Chapter 8), the herpes simplex virus (HSV-1) may cause a systemic illness with extensive mouth ulceration when first encountered.

History

- Usually a child under 5 years
- Short history of fever and malaise
- May be refusing to eat or drink

Examination

- Temperature
- Check for dehydration
- Enlarged cervical lymph nodes (especially submandibular)
- Multiple small ulcers on tongue, palate and buccal mucosa (cheek lining)

Self-care

- Ensure adequate fluid intake (a straw or very cold drinks may help)
- Use paracetamol[P] for pain relief
- Benzydamine spray (e.g. Difflam® OTC) may be helpful
- Apply Vaseline® to lips
- Take precautions to reduce infection spread
- Avoid contact with babies aged under 4 weeks

Prescription

- Offer oral aciclovir if onset <3 days

Reference

Goldman, R.D. 2016. Acyclovir for herpetic gingivostomatitis in children. *Can Fam Physician*; 62(5),403–404.

'SWOLLEN GLANDS' (ENLARGED CERVICAL LYMPH NODES)

History

- Sore throat, earache or rashes
- Fever
- Other symptoms
- Duration of swelling
- 🚩 Night sweats
- 🚩 Weight loss
- 🚩 Recurrent infections
- 🚩 Unexplained bruising
- 🚩 Progressive enlargement over time (if present more than 3 weeks)

Examination

- Temperature
- Location, number and size of enlarged nodes
- Local tenderness or heat
- Throat – any inflammation or exudate

Tests (if symptoms last more than 3 weeks)

- FBC, CRP
- Paul Bunnell/Monospot if aged 15–25
- Consider HIV test

Self-care advice

- Explain that the glands are the body's defence against infection
- Can use ibuprofen[P] or paracetamol if pain is severe
- Worsening advice: seek help if not settling after 3 weeks

RED FLAGS

Refer to senior colleague if:
- Night sweats or weight loss (*possible serious systemic infection or malignant process*)
- Single very large painful node or one enlarging rapidly (*may contain an abscess*)
- Node >2 cm in size (*unlikely to be a normal reaction to infection*)
- Supraclavicular node (*may be sign of malignancy*)
- Lymph nodes which are hard, fixed or enlarging progressively over 3–6 weeks (*may be a sign of HIV, lymphoma, leukaemia, sarcoidosis or tuberculosis*)
- Recurrent infections (*may be a sign of HIV or leukaemia*) or unexplained bruising (*may be a sign of leukaemia*)

Reference

Tidy, C. 2017. Generalised lymphadenopathy. Patient+. patient.info/doctor/generalised-lymphadenopathy.

MUMPS

A viral infection of the salivary glands. This was previously a disease of children that had become rare following the introduction of mumps vaccination. Most cases are without serious consequence, but complications include orchitis/oophoritis, pancreatitis, viral meningitis and risk of miscarriage between 12–16 weeks' gestation. In 2005, because of the unfounded measles, mumps and rubella (MMR) vaccine scare, there was a large increase in mumps cases in the 15–24 age group. It is a notifiable disease.

History

- Vaccination history
- Contact with mumps (up to 28 days before)
- Swelling/pain of parotid glands, worse on chewing
- Dry mouth, making it harder to swallow
- Fever
- Malaise
- Headache
- Earache
- Abdominal or testicular pain
- ⚑ Drowsiness/photophobia/vomiting/severe headache

Examination

- Temperature
- Parotid glands (swelling may be unilateral or bilateral)
- Earlobe may be pushed upward and outward
- ⚑ Neck stiffness, photophobia, confusion/drowsiness

Tests

- Confirmation of the diagnosis (using a special salivary sample kit) may be requested by the Health Protection Team (HPT) after the disease has been notified

Self-care

- Paracetamol or ibuprofen[P] may ease the discomfort
- Maintain fluid intake
- Acidic fruit juices may intensify the pain and should be avoided
- Infectious from 2 days before, to 5 days after, the onset of swelling
- Vulnerable contacts (who have not previously received two doses of mumps vaccine) should be vaccinated. Unfortunately, vaccination will not give immediate protection
- Worsening advice: seek help if severe headache, vomiting, neck stiffness, photophobia, abdominal or testicular pain

RED FLAG

- Symptoms of meningitis or encephalitis (*may include severe headache, vomiting, neck stiffness, photophobia, confusion, drowsiness; admit under Medical or Paediatrics*)

EAR PROBLEMS

History
- Duration and type of pain/discomfort
- Fever
- Hearing impairment
- Discharge
- Previous ear problems/perforation
- Any previous treatment
- 🚩 Immunosuppressed

Examination
- Temperature
- If feverish, view ear from behind to look for outward and downward displacement of pinna (due to mastoiditis) and check mastoid area for tenderness and swelling
- Use an otoscope to check:
  - Ear canal for inflammation, foreign body, discharge or swelling (generalised or local, for example, boil). Pain on insertion of the otoscope suggests inflammation of the external canal
  - Tympanic membrane to assess colour, dullness, perforation, bulging/retraction and fluid level

Differential diagnosis
The most likely causes of acute earache are otitis media, otitis externa, boil in the ear canal, hard wax or Eustachian tube dysfunction.

Reference
van den Aardweg, M.T., Rovers, M.M., de Ru, J.A., Albers, F.W., and Schilder, A.G. 2008. A systematic review of diagnostic criteria for acute mastoiditis in children. *Otology & Neurotology*; 29(6):751–757. doi: 10.1097/MAO.0b013e31817f736b

OTITIS MEDIA

Otitis media is commonest in small children, though it may occur in adults. It causes pain, deafness and sometimes fever, vomiting and loss of balance. The eardrum is red. It may be bulging, or discharge may be present. If the history is suggestive but the drum cannot be seen (e.g. because of wax), it is safest to assume that otitis media is present. Pink eardrums are to be expected in fever if other membranes are inflamed (e.g. conjunctivitis, red throat), and during/after crying.

Self-care
- Recommend ibuprofen[P] or paracetamol at maximum dose for age to treat the pain
- Explain that antibiotics are not helpful for most patients with otitis media. 60% of patients will be pain-free within 24 hours, whether or not they take antibiotics, and the chance of experiencing a side effect from the antibiotic is greater than the chance of benefiting
- Flying or diving may cause severe pain and even perforation and should be avoided while pain is present
- Severe infections may cause temporary deafness by perforation of the eardrum, which will usually heal in 2 weeks
- Reassure that ear infections very rarely cause permanent hearing damage

Prescription (only if indicated – see Box 5.3)
- Amoxicillin at maximum dose for age for 5–7 days (500 mg three times daily for adults)
- If allergic to penicillin, give clarithromycin[PIQ] (500 mg twice daily for adults)
- If not responding to amoxicillin within 3 days, change to co-amoxiclav (500/125 mg three times daily for adults)

Action: See Box 5.3

 BOX 5.3 ANTIBIOTICS FOR OTITIS MEDIA

Prescribe an antibiotic if:

- Seriously ill
- Prolonged and worsening
- Immunosuppressed
- Symptoms >3 days and not improving

Consider an antibiotic if:

- Child younger than 2 years with bilateral otitis media
- Child younger than 3 years with severe bulging of tympanic membrane (Tähtinen, 2017)
- Child with perforation and discharge

In a child with grommets and ear discharge, topical antibiotic/steroid drops (e.g. Cilodex®) are more effective than oral antibiotics (Steele, 2017).
    N.B. There is little evidence on the role of antibiotics in adults with otitis media.

 RED FLAGS

- Suspected mastoiditis (*refer same day to ENT*)
- Immunosuppressed patient with hearing loss, pain and discharge (*if not responding to treatment within 72 hours; refer same day to ENT*)
- If hearing does not return to normal within 14 days (*may need ENT outpatient referral for monitoring of perforation*)
- Persistent foul-smelling discharge and hearing loss (*possible cholesteatoma; refer to ENT outpatients*)

References

NICE CKS. 2015. Otitis media – acute. cks.nice.org.uk/otitis-media-acute.

NICE NG91. 2018. Otitis media (acute): Antimicrobial prescribing. www.nice.org.uk/guidance/ng91.

NICE NG98. 2018. Hearing loss in adults: Assessment and management. www.nice.org.uk/guidance/ng98.

Steele, D.W., Adam, G., Di, M., Halladay, C.W., Balk, E.M., and Trikalinos, T.A. 2017. Prevention and treatment of tympanostomy tube otorrhea: A meta-analysis. *Pediatrics*; p.e20170667.

Tähtinen, P.A., Laine, M.K., and Ruohola, A. 2017. Prognostic factors for treatment failure in acute otitis media. *Pediatrics*; 140(3):e20170072.

Venekamp, R.P., Sanders, S.L., Glasziou, P.P., Del Mar, C.B., and Rovers, M.M. 2015. Antibiotics for acute otitis media in children. *Cochrane Database Syst Rev*; (6). Art. No.: CD000219. doi: 10.1002/14651858.CD000219.pub4.

OTITIS EXTERNA

This is a form of infected eczema that causes itchy discomfort rather than pain. It may follow inappropriate probing of the ear with a hairgrip or cotton bud or the presence of a foreign body. Insertion of the otoscope is often uncomfortable. The canal looks irregular, red or moist, perhaps with discharge. It can be recurrent, often with secondary fungal infection occurring after initial antibiotic treatment. The most common pathogens are Pseudomonas (20%–60%) and Staphylococcus (10%–70%), which may co-exist. The treatment for otitis externa may vary depending on the presence of perforation of the tympanic membrane or grommets (see Box 5.4).

Test

- Consider taking a swab if there is copious discharge, resistant or recurrent infection, but results may be misleading – remember that the sensitivity data relate to oral antibiotics, and topical treatment gives higher concentrations

Self-care advice

- Avoid putting anything into the ear canal (remember the old adage 'put nothing smaller than your elbow in your ear!')
- Use cotton wool and Vaseline® to keep shampoo and shower gel out of inflamed ears while showering or washing hair
- Dry inside ears with hairdryer on lowest setting

- Use ear plugs when swimming. Avoid swimming while ear is inflamed
- Use acetic acid spray (Earcalm® OTC) before swimming, after swimming, at bedtime, and at the first sign of irritation

---

BOX 5.4 IS THE TYMPANIC MEMBRANE PERFORATED?

If the tympanic membrane cannot be seen (e.g. due to wax in canal), then suspect perforation if:

- Patient can taste medication placed in the ear, *or*
- Patient can blow air out of the ear when the nose is pinched, *or*
- Grommet inserted in the past year (and not known to have fallen out)

Prescription

- Acetic acid spray (e.g. Earcalm®C) for mild infections (administered directly into each affected ear at least three times daily: morning, evening, and after swimming, showering, or bathing. Maximum dosage frequency one spray every 2–3 hours)
- If very inflamed, offer eardrops containing an antibiotic and a corticosteroid for 7–14 days. They should be warmed to room temperature before use. All antibiotic drops except Cilodex®PC are contraindicated if there is a grommet or perforated eardrum (see Box 5.4). They contain aminoglycoside antibiotics, whereas Cilodex® contains ciprofloxacin. In other situations there is little evidence to inform the choice; be guided by their price and availability. Options include:
  - Gentisone HC®P, containing gentamicin (apply two to four drops four to five times a day, including a dose at bedtime)
  - Sofradex®P, containing framycetin and gramicidin (apply four to six times a day; may be administered every 30–60 minutes in severe conditions until controlled, then reduce frequency)
  - Cilodex®PC, containing ciprofloxacin (apply four drops twice daily for 7 days)
- If unable to use eardrops, use Otomize®PC spray, which contains neomycin (one spray three times a day for adults and children over 2 years)
- If swab shows a fungal cause (around 10% of otitis externa cases), then first try clotrimazole 1% solution two to three times a day continued for 2 weeks after the infection appears to have cleared. Treatment may be needed for up to a few months. Occasionally, oral antifungal treatment is needed

Action: See Box 5.5

 BOX 5.5 ORAL ANTIBIOTICS FOR OTITIS EXTERNA

Topical antibiotic is preferred. Prescribe an oral antibiotic only if:

- Canal completely blocked with debris and suction not available
- Signs of systemic infection
- Cellulitis
- Immunosuppressed
- Diabetes

Oral antibiotic choice

- Flucloxacillin for 7 days (250–500 mg four times daily for adults)
- If patient is allergic to penicillin, give clarithromycin[PIQ] (250 mg twice daily for adults)
- These oral antibiotics will not treat Pseudomonas infection. If swab shows Pseudomonas and topical treatment is ineffective, or the patient is at high risk, use dual therapy with topical Cilodex®PC and oral ciprofloxacin[PCIQ] (500 mg two times daily for adults)

 RED FLAGS

- Severe infection in high-risk patient with diabetes or immunosuppression (*'malignant' otitis externa extending into bone; same-day referral to ENT*)
- Canal completely occluded or persistent/recurrent symptoms (*referral for microsuction according to local protocol*)

References

Knott, L. 2017. Fungal ear infection (otomycosis). Patient.info. patient.info/doctor/fungal-ear-infection-otomycosis.

NICE CKS. 2016. Otitis externa. cks.nice.org.uk/otitis-externa.

Rosenfeld, R.M., Schwartz, S.R., Cannon, C.R., Roland, P.R., Simon, G.R., Kaparaboyna, A.K., Huang, W.W. et al. 2014. Clinical practice guideline: Acute otitis externa. *Otolaryngol. – Head Neck Surg*; 150 (1 Suppl): s1–24. http://journals.sagepub.com/doi/full/10.1177/0194599813517083.

Walton, L. 2012. Otitis externa. *BMJ*; 344:e3623. doi: 10.1136/bmj.e3623.

BOIL IN EAR CANAL

This causes a localised red swelling in the canal, often with unilateral deafness. Introduce the otoscope gradually and gently, looking through it as you do this because impacting the earpiece directly on to a boil can cause severe pain.

Self-care

- Take paracetamol or ibuprofen[P] to relieve the pain
- The ear may discharge

Action: See Box 5.6

 BOX 5.6 ANTIBIOTICS FOR BOIL IN EAR CANAL

Prescribe an antibiotic if:

- Cellulitis spreading to pinna
- Fever
- Immunosuppressed
- Diabetes

Antibiotic choice

- Flucloxacillin for 7 days (250–500 mg four times daily for adults)
- If patient is allergic to penicillin, give clarithromycin[PIQ] (250 mg twice daily for adults)

Reference

NICE CKS. 2016. Otitis externa. cks.nice.org.uk/otitis-externa#!scenario.

EUSTACHIAN TUBE DYSFUNCTION

This may follow an episode of otitis media or upper respiratory tract infection (URTI). It is commoner in children. The hearing is impaired, and the ear is intermittently uncomfortable. The sufferer may describe sometimes feeling like they are 'underwater' or 'on a plane'. The eardrum may appear normal, retracted or bulging. A fluid level may be seen behind the drum, which is not inflamed.

Self-care

- Explain that the eardrum is a sensitive structure that hurts when pressure changes. When catarrh blocks the Eustachian tube, changes in atmospheric pressure cause earache that comes and goes
- Nasal decongestant drops or sprays, for example, Otrivine®[PC], for no more than 3 days (two to three drops or one spray up to three times a day). They are licensed for 7 days' use but see Wallace et al. (2008)
- Carefully 'pop' the ears by trying to breathe out with mouth closed and nostrils shut (pinching the nose). Yawning and swallowing can also help
- If these manoeuvres fail, an Otovent® balloon (available OTC) may be tried to open the Eustachian tube
- Paracetamol or ibuprofen[P] may ease the discomfort

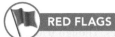

RED FLAGS

- Rapid-onset unilateral hearing loss without visible cause (*urgent referral to ENT outpatients to exclude acoustic neuroma*)
- Not resolved after 6 weeks (*may need ENT outpatient referral*)

References

Edmiston, R., and Mitchell, C. 2013. Hearing loss in adults. *BMJ*; 346:f2496. doi: 10.1136/bmj.f2496. *Red flag evidence.*

Wallace, D.V., and Dykeqic, M.S. 2008. The diagnosis and management of rhinitis: An updated practice parameter. *J Allerg Clin Immunol*; 122(2):S1–S84. www.aaaai.org/Aaaai/media/MediaLibrary/PDF%20Documents/Practice%20and%20Parameters/rhinitis2008-diagnosis-management.pdf. *Rebound congestion may develop within 3 days of use of topical decongestants.*

EAR WAX

Wax is a mixture of several substances including dead skin cells, cerumen (produced by special glands in the ear canal) and sebum from sebaceous glands. It is mildly acidic and antibacterial. The gradual migration of cells in the ear canal causes wax to travel, assisted by jaw movement, towards the outside of the ear over a few weeks, so it cleans and protects the delicate surfaces.

History

- Deafness
- Ear discomfort/blockage
- Tinnitus
- Itching
- Use of cotton buds
- History of perforation

Examination

Note extent of wax and whether it is impacted against tympanic membrane.

Self-care

- Do not insert cotton buds inside the ear canal
- Use olive oil ear drops, at body temperature, three times daily for at least five days
- The use of ear candles is not supported by evidence

Action

If self-care is ineffective, consider microsuction (preferred) or irrigation. Contraindications to irrigation include:

- Perforation of the tympanic membrane. Some ENT specialists may permit irrigation if there is an old healed perforation, but this should be agreed in advance
- Grommets
- Previous ear surgery
- Discharge from ear in the previous 12 months
- Otitis media in the previous 6 weeks
- Cleft palate, even after surgical correction
- Current otitis externa
- Foreign body in the ear
- Previous problem with irrigation

References

McGrath, P. 2014. Secretion secrets: Things you didn't know about ear wax. BBC News. www.bbc.co.uk/news/health-26527266.

NICE CKS. 2016. Earwax. cks.nice.org.uk/earwax.

COMMON COLD (CORYZA)

A mild, self-limiting upper respiratory tract infection (URTI) caused by a wide range of different viruses. Though usually associated with a dry cough, even a productive cough with green phlegm is most likely viral (in people without COPD).

History
- Duration
- Sore throat
- Blocked or discharging nose, sneezing
- Hoarse voice
- Cough
- Joint and muscle pain
- Fever
- Immunosuppressed

Examination
- Temperature
- Throat (usually appears normal)
- Cervical lymph nodes
- Ears
- Chest

Self-care
- Paracetamol or ibuprofen[P] if needed for sore throat/headache/body pains
- Gargling with salt water (half a teaspoon of salt in 250 ml water)
- Honey (if aged over 12 months) and lemon
- Sodium chloride nasal drops (for babies) or spray (e.g. Sterimar Hypertonic®)
- Chlorphenamine[PBI] (4 mg at bedtime, repeated after 4 hours if necessary, for adults) at night may help congestion and aid sleep
- Nasal decongestant drops or sprays, for example, Otrivine®[PC], for no more than 3 days (two to three drops or one spray up to three times a day)
- Expect resolution in 7 days (adults) or 14 days (children)
- Some evidence suggests that high-dose zinc and vitamin C may shorten the duration of colds. However, the most effective doses of zinc and vitamin C are above those licensed for sale over the counter
- Frequent handwashing and avoiding sharing towels and toys may reduce the spread of infection

Although steam inhalation has been recommended as a home remedy for many years, there is no evidence of benefit, and children are at risk of serious burns.

References

Al Himdani, S., Javed, M.U., Hughes, J., Falconer, O., Bidder, C., Hemington-Gorse, S., and Nguyen, D. 2016. Home remedy or hazard? Management and costs of paediatric steam inhalation therapy burn injuries. *Br J Gen Pract*; 66(644):e193–e199. doi: 10.3399/bjgp16X684289.

Deckx, L., De Sutter, A.I.M., Guo, L., Mir, N.A., and van Driel, M.L. 2016. Nasal decongestants in monotherapy for the common cold. *Cochrane Database Syst Rev*; (10). Art. No.: CD009612. doi: 10.1002/14651858.CD009612.pub2.

Hemilä, H. 2017. Vitamin C and infections. *Nutrients*; 9(4):E339. doi: 10.3390/nu9040339.

Hemilä, H., Petrus, E.J., Fitzgerald, J.T., and Prasad, A. 2016. Zinc acetate lozenges for treating the common cold: An individual patient data meta-analysis. *Br J Clin Pharmacol*; 82:1393–1398. doi: 10.1111/bcp.13057.

Karsch-Völk, M., Barrett, B., Kiefer, D., Bauer, R., Ardjomand-Woelkart, K., and Linde, K. 2014. Echinacea for preventing and treating the common cold. *Cochrane Database Syst Rev*, Issue 2. Art. No.: CD000530. doi: 10.1002/14651858.CD000530.pub3.

Paul, I.M., Beiler, J.S., King, T.S., Clapp, E.R., Vallati, J., and Berlin, C.M. 2010. Vapor rub, petrolatum, and no treatment for children with nocturnal cough and cold symptoms. *Pediatrics*; 126(6):1092–1099.

Public Health England. 2013. Green phlegm and snot 'not always a sign of an infection needing antibiotics'. www.gov.uk/government/news/green-phlegm-and-snot-not-always-a-sign-of-an-infection-needing-antibiotics.

Singh, M., and Singh, M. 2013. Heated, humidified air for the common cold. *Cochrane Database Syst Rev*; (6). Art. No.: CD001728. doi: 10.1002/14651858.CD001728.pub5.

Wallace, D.V., and Dykeqic, M.S. 2008. The diagnosis and management of rhinitis: An updated practice parameter. *J Allerg Clin Immunol*; 122(2):S1–S84. www.aaaai.org/Aaaai/media/MediaLibrary/PDF%20Documents/Practice%20and%20Parameters/rhinitis2008-diagnosis-management.pdf. *Rebound congestion may develop within 3 days of use of topical decongestants.*

SINUSITIS

This condition is very difficult to diagnose because the traditional symptoms and signs are unreliable. It is usually viral.

History

- Duration – average 18–20 days
- Nasal blockage
- Purulent nasal discharge
- Facial pain, typically worse on bending forward
- Toothache
- Visual disturbance
- Fever
- 🚩 Immunosuppressed

Examination

Although there is often tenderness over the sinuses, there are no reliable diagnostic signs of sinusitis. To make sure the infection is not more generalised check:

- Temperature
- Throat (look for post-nasal discharge)
- Ears
- 🚩 Localised swelling or redness anywhere on the face

Self-care

- Avoid smoky atmospheres
- Use a sinus rinse kit available OTC (e.g. NeilMed Sinus Rinse®) or irrigate the nose with sodium chloride solution (e.g. Sterimar Hypertonic®)
- Warm face packs
- Analgesia with paracetamol or ibuprofen[P] if needed
- Decongestant nasal drops or spray, for example, Otrivine®[PC] (for no more than three days)

Prescription

- Consider high-dose nasal corticosteroid, for example, beclometasone[PC] (100 mcg twice daily into each nostril, reduced to 50 mcg twice daily when symptoms controlled)
- Antibiotic only if indicated (see Box 5.7)

 BOX 5.7 ANTIBIOTICS FOR SINUSITIS

Prescribe an antibiotic if:

- Seriously ill
- Immunosuppressed
- Prolonged and worsening symptoms >10 days *or*
- Purulent discharge and severe local pain (particularly if unilateral)

Antibiotic Choice

Adults

- Phenoxymethylpenicillin for 5 days (500 mg four times daily)
- If allergic to penicillin, use doxycycline[PBC] (200 mg on the first day then 100 mg once daily, 5 days in total) or clarithromycin[PIQ] (250 mg twice daily for 5 days)
- If systemically unwell, at a high risk of complications, or worsening symptoms despite 2-3 days of the first-line antibiotic, use co-amoxiclav (500/125 mg three times daily for 5 days) or azithromycin[PQ] for 3 days (500 mg once daily for adults)

Children

- Phenoxymethylpenicillin for 5 days. An alternative if the child cannot tolerate the taste of phenoxymethylpenicillin suspension is amoxicillin
- If allergic to penicillin, use clarithromycin[PIQ] for 5 days
- If systemically unwell, at a high risk of complications, or worsening symptoms despite 2–3 days of the first-line antibiotic, use co-amoxiclav for 5 days or azithromycin[PQ] for 3 days

> **RED FLAGS**
>
> - Eye symptoms, for example, periorbital oedema, double vision, reduced visual acuity (*intraorbital complications; refer to ENT same day*)
> - Severe frontal headache or swelling over frontal bone (*intracranial complications; admit under ENT*)
> - Localised swelling or redness anywhere on the face (*possible cellulitis; refer same-day to ENT*)

References

Lemiengre, M.B., van Driel, M.L., Merenstein, D., Young, J., and De Sutter, A.I.M. 2012. Antibiotics for clinically diagnosed acute rhinosinusitis in adults. *Cochrane Database Syst Rev*; (10). Art. No.: CD006089. doi: 10.1002/14651858.CD006089.pub4.

Little, P., Stuart, B., Mullee, M., Thoma,s T., Johnson, S., Leydon, G. et al. 2016. Effectiveness of steam inhalation and nasal irrigation for chronic or recurrent sinus symptoms in primary care: A pragmatic randomized controlled trial. *CMAJ*; 188(13):940–949. doi: 10.1503/cmaj.160362. *Steam inhalations were not effective, but nasal irrigation provided some symptom relief.*

NICE NG79. 2017. Sinusitis (acute): Antimicrobial prescribing. www.nice.org.uk/guidance/ng79.

Ramey, J.T., Bailen, E., and Lockey, R.F. 2006. Rhinitis medicamentosa. *J Investig Allergol Clin Immunol*; 16(3):148.

Zalmanovici, T.A., and Yaphe, J. 2013. Intranasal steroids for acute sinusitis. *Cochrane Database Syst Rev*; (12). Art. No.: CD005149. doi: 10.1002/14651858.CD005149.pub4.

HAY FEVER

History

- Seasonal (usually April to August)
- Frequent sneezing
- Blocked nose
- Red, itchy, watery eyes
- Dry, sore throat
- Wheeze, chest tightness, cough
- Any treatment tried already?
- If so, with what effect?

Examination

- Check eyes for discharge (suggests infection)
- Check nose for polyps

Self-care

Pollen grains are very, very small, so avoidance is impossible. Advice can only aim to reduce the exposure to high concentrations. Some form of treatment for residual symptoms is necessary for most people.

- Avoid long grass, fragrant flowers and newly mowed lawns

- When choosing a car, consider one with a pollen filter

- There is no evidence to support the standard advice to sleep with windows closed

- Patients and parents can access useful information about hay fever and other allergic conditions at www.itchysneezywheezy.co.uk

- Nasal irrigation with saline is effective for children, though often unpopular

- Oral antihistamines such as loratadine or cetirizine (OTC, 10 mg once daily for adults) reduce all hay fever symptoms, but even non-drowsy preparations may not be permitted for people in safety-critical occupations

- There is no evidence that one antihistamine is more effective than others overall, but individual patients may differ in their response, and there are important differences in the unwanted effects. Avoid antihistamines known to cause sedation (e.g. chlorphenamine[PBI]) where this is not needed. Modern drugs are far less likely to cause drowsiness, but cetirizine is slightly more likely to do so than others

- Steroid nasal sprays (OTC) reduce nasal symptoms more than oral antihistamines but have no proven effect on eye symptoms. They are more effective if started a few days (ideally two weeks) before symptoms are expected to begin. These are not available OTC for treating children (at the time of publication). Their benefits will be reduced if they are not used correctly; see Figure 5.1. They may be used in pregnancy and breastfeeding, but a prescription will be required

- Decongestant nasal sprays (e.g. Otrivine®[PC], OTC, two to three drops or one spray up to three times a day for adults) can provide quick relief for adults and children over 6 years but should not be used more than 3 days as they can cause rebound symptoms

- Sodium cromoglicate eyedrops (OTC, four times daily) can be bought as an additional treatment (but a prescription will be needed if pregnant or breastfeeding), but they are slow to take effect. These may sting, especially if the eyes are already inflamed, and should be started at least 1 week before the season. Otrivine Antistin®[PBC] drops (OTC, two to three times daily) are faster acting but should not be used for more than 3 days because of their vasoconstrictor effect (Table 5.1)

Prescriptions (Figure 5.1, Table 5.1)

- Antihistamine: there is little role for prescribing oral antihistamines as they are available OTC (for much less than a prescription charge). NHS England issued guidance to CCGs in 2018 advising against such prescriptions for mild/moderate hay fever. Loratadine is available OTC for children over 2 years. Oral antihistamines should therefore only be prescribed in exceptional circumstances (e.g. pregnancy or breastfeeding; cetirizine has the best safety record, but aim to avoid prescribing any drugs in the first trimester)

- Nasal symptoms: adults with mild/moderate hay fever should obtain a steroid nasal spray OTC. A prescription will be needed if treating a child. There is concern that beclomethasone[PC] or fluticasone[C] may slow growth in children (Lee et al., 2014; Passali et al., 2016); instead use mometasone[C] for children over 3 years. Consider the nasal antihistamine azelastine[PBC] (Rhinolast®[PBC]) 1 spray twice daily into each nostril if symptoms are infrequent, as it has a quicker onset than nasal steroids and can be used 'as required'. It is licensed for use in children over 6 years

- Eye symptoms: topical antihistamine eye drops of azelastine[PBC] (apply twice daily, increased if necessary to four times a day) are quicker acting but less effective than sodium cromoglicate eyedrops (OTC) and are only available with a prescription

- If usual treatment ineffective, consider trying:
  - Montelukast[PB] (as effective as antihistamines in children)
  - Ranitidine (*unlicensed indication*) 150mg twice daily for adults (for more information, see the Members' section of the NMIC website)
  - Fluticasone/azelastine[PBC] nasal spray (Dymista®[PBC], 1 spray twice daily into each nostril)

- In severe cases, prednisolone[IP] for 7 days (15–20 mg daily for adults, 5–10 mg daily for children) (Figure 5.2)

For nasal sprays (see Figure 5.1):

- Shake bottle well
- Look down
- Using RIGHT hand for LEFT nostril, put nozzle just inside nose aiming straight in, towards the back of the head, and towards outside wall
- Squirt once or twice (two different directions)
- Change hands and repeat for other side
- DO NOT SNIFF HARD

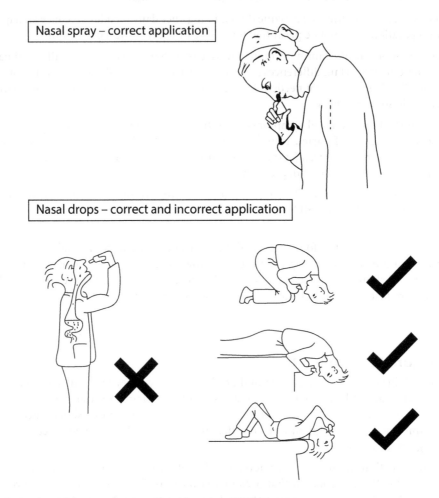

Nasal spray – correct application

Nasal drops – correct and incorrect application

Figure 5.1 The correct use of nasal drops and sprays. (Scadding et al., 2008.)

Table 5.1 Recommended medication for hay fever

Hay fever medication	Over the counter	Prescription
Steroid nasal spray	Whichever is best value	Beclometasone[PC] (adult) Mometasone[C] (child ≥6y)
Decongestant nasal spray	Whichever is best value	Oxymetazoline[C]
Antihistamine – oral	Whichever is best value	Loratadine Cetirizine
Antihistamine – eye (for short-term symptom relief)	Otrivine Antistin®[PBC] for no more than 3 days (child ≥12y)	Azelastine[PBC] (child ≥4y)
Long-term eyedrop	Sodium cromoglicate	Sodium cromoglicate

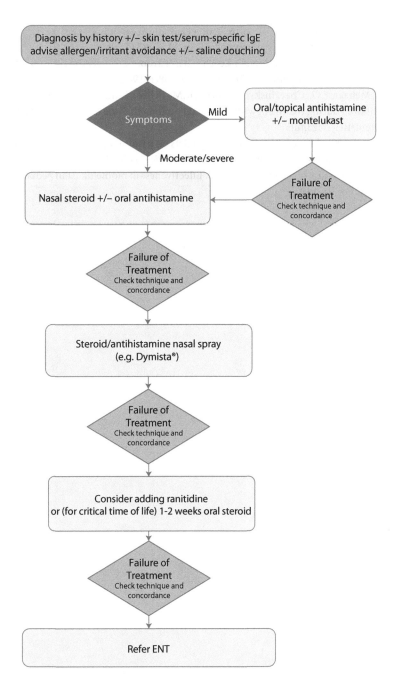

Figure 5.2 Management of allergic rhinitis in adults. (Adapted from Lipworth, B. et al. 2017.)

References

Barr, J.G., Al-Reefy, H., Fox, A.T., and Hopkins, C. 2014. Allergic rhinitis in children. *BMJ*; 349:g4153 doi: 10.1136/bmj.g4153. *Evidence for saline irrigation and montelukast.*

Lee, L.A., Sterling, R., Máspero, J., Clements, D., Ellsworth, A., Pedersen, S. 2014. Growth velocity reduced with once-daily fluticasone furoate nasal spray in prepubescent children with perennial allergic rhinitis. *The Journal of Allergy and Clinical Immunology: In Practice*; 2(4):421–7. www.sciencedirect.com/science/article/pii/S221321981400172X.

Lipworth, B., Newton, J., Ram, B., Small, I., and Schwarze, J. 2017. An algorithm recommendation for the pharmacological management of allergic rhinitis in the UK: a consensus statement from an expert panel. *npj Prim Care Respir Med*; 27, Article number: 3. doi: 10.1038/s41533-016-0001-y. *Suggested order of trying different treatments.*

Meltzer, E.O., Tripathy, I., Máspero, J.F., Wu, W., and Philpot, E. 2009. Safety and tolerability of fluticasone furoate nasal spray once daily in paediatric patients aged 6-11 years with allergic rhinitis: subanalysis of three randomized, double-blind, placebo-controlled, multicentre studies. *Clin Drug Investig*; 29:79–86. doi: 10.2165/0044011-200929020-00002.

Passali, D., Spinosi, M.C., Crisanti, A., Bellussi, L.M. 2016. Mometasone furoate nasal spray: a systematic review. *Multidisciplinary Respiratory Medicine*; 11:18. www.ncbi.nlm.nih.gov/pmc/articles/PMC4852427/.

Scadding, G.K., Durham, S.R., Mirakian, R., Jones, N.S., Leech, S.C., Farooque, S., Ryan, D. et al. 2008. BSACI guidelines for the management of allergic and non-allergic rhinitis. *Clin Exp Allergy*; 38(1):19–42.

Skoner, D.P., Rachelefsky, G.S., Meltzer, E.O., Chervinsky, P., Morris, R.M., Seltzer, J.M., Storms, W.W., and Wood, R.A. 2000. Detection of growth suppression in children during treatment with intranasal beclomethasone dipropionate. *Pediatrics*; 105(2). http://pediatrics.aappublications.org/content/105/2/e23.full.

Wang, D., Clement, P., and Smitz, J. 1996. Effect of H1 and H2 antagonists on nasal symptoms and mediator release in atopic patients after nasal allergen challenge during the pollen season. *Acta Otolaryngologica*; 116(1):91–96. doi: 10.3109/00016489609137720.

Yilmaz, O., Altintas, D., Rondon, C., Cingi, C., and Oghan, F. 2013. Effectiveness of montelukast in pediatric patients with allergic rhinitis. *Int J Pediatr Otorhinolaryngol*; 77(12):1922–1924.

CHAPTER 6

Eyes

SORE OR RED EYES

History

- Duration
- Associated upper respiratory tract infection (URTI) or rhinitis
- Bilateral or unilateral
- Discharge
- Pattern of symptoms (worse outdoors suggests allergic conjunctivitis, worse after computer work suggests dry eyes)
- Treatment already tried
- ⚑ Any problem with vision
- ⚑ Pain or photophobia
- ⚑ History of trauma/foreign body/drilling or grinding, especially metal
- ⚑ Contact lens use
- ⚑ Previous eye problems, such as iritis
- ⚑ Background of autoimmune conditions, such as inflammatory bowel disease or ankylosing spondylitis

Examination

A magnifying glass and a light may be helpful, but an ophthalmoscope examination is not needed. In uncomplicated conjunctivitis, examination may be unnecessary.

- Normal visual acuity is the most helpful sign in excluding a serious eye condition. If the patient is unable to confirm this, check with a Snellen chart (they should wear their usual glasses for this, if applicable)
- Check eyelids (stye, meibomian cyst, cellulitis)
- Examine roots of eyelashes for scales (blepharitis)
- Look for spots on the surrounding skin (shingles)
- Discharge
- Redness – diffuse or localised
- Pupil shape and responsiveness to light
- Look for foreign body (evert eyelid), especially if symptoms unilateral

Test

- Stain with fluorescein if unilateral symptoms or history of trauma (but ensure any contact lens is removed first)

Action – depends on cause

1. Infective conjunctivitis
2. Blepharitis
3. Allergic conjunctivitis
4. Dry eyes
5. Stye
6. Meibomian cyst
7. Corneal ulcer

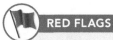

RED FLAGS

- Reduced visual acuity (*possible corneal ulcer, iritis or acute glaucoma; refer to Ophthalmology*)
- Pain, not gritty discomfort (*possible corneal ulcer; refer to Ophthalmology*)
- Photophobia (*possible iritis or corneal ulcer; refer to Ophthalmology*)
- Previous serious eye disease or background of autoimmune disease (*possible iritis; refer to Ophthalmology*)
- Baby under 4 weeks with red eye/s (*possible chlamydia or gonorrhoea; refer to Ophthalmology*)
- Possible metallic or glass foreign body, or high-speed injury (*refer A&E, even if no external abnormality*)
- Contact lens wearer (*possible keratitis; refer to Ophthalmology. Ask patient to take lens and cleaning solution to appointment*)
- Severe inflammation, especially around cornea (*possible corneal ulcer or iritis; refer to Ophthalmology*)
- Any abnormality seen using fluorescein (*possible corneal ulcer; refer to Ophthalmology*)
- Irregular pupil or non-reactive (*possible iritis or acute glaucoma; refer to Ophthalmology*)
- Facial shingles (*possible corneal ulcer; refer to Ophthalmology*)

INFECTIVE CONJUNCTIVITIS

Sore eyes, red conjunctival membranes, usually with discharge. Most cases are viral: in children only 10% are caused by bacteria (Chen et al., 2017). May be unilateral, especially in early stages. Check for scales on roots of eyelashes; if present, see section on *Blepharitis*.

Self-care

- Should settle without treatment in 1–2 weeks
- Clean discharge away with cotton wool soaked in cooled boiled water
- Remove contact lenses, if worn, until problem has completely settled
- Lubricant eye drops such as hypromellose or Viscotears® may reduce discomfort
- Viral conjunctivitis is very likely if associated URTI
- Chloramphenicol[PB] makes little difference to comfort or speed of recovery and should not be used unless symptoms are severe, for example, the eyelids stuck together with thick discharge
- At best, topical antibiotic may shorten the illness by 0.3 days (NNT 13; Jefferis et al., 2011); up to 10% of people treated with chloramphenicol[PB] suffer adverse reactions
- If used, chloramphenicol[PB] eyedrops should be applied as often as possible (every 2 hours ideally initially). If severe, apply ointment at night also (treat only the infected eye/s). On the rare occasions when chloramphenicol is needed it should be obtained OTC (unless patient aged under 2 years)
- Wash hands after touching eyes, use own face cloth, makeup, pillowcase and towel. If used, mascara and eyeliner may carry bacteria
- Schools and nurseries often prefer that children with conjunctivitis do not attend until the discharge has gone. Public Health England does not recommend exclusion, and topical antibiotics do not reduce the infective period. The Royal College of GPs (RCGP) wrote to Ofsted about this issue in 2016
- Complications are rare, but urgently seek advice if:
  - Severe eye pain or photophobia
  - Visual problems
  - Eye redness becomes severe

Action/prescription

- None for most
- Chloramphenicol[PB] is not available over the counter (OTC) for children aged under 2 years, so if it is indicated, then a prescription should be issued. Ointment may be easier to apply in babies
- Avoid chloramphenicol if:
  - History of bone marrow problem, for example aplastic anaemia (use ofloxacin[PBQ] instead)
  - Pregnancy and lactation (use sodium fusidate, but narrow-spectrum)

References

Chen, F.V., Chang, T.C., and Cavuoto, K.M. 2017. Patient demographic and microbiology trends in bacterial conjunctivitis in children. *J AAPOS*; Dec 2017:66.

Finnikin, S., and Jolly, K. 2016. Nursery sickness policies and their influence on prescribing for conjunctivitis: Audit and questionnaire survey. *Br J Gen Pract*; 66(650):e674–e679.

Jefferis, J., Perera, R., Everitt, H., van Weert, H., Rietveld, R., Glasziou, P., and Rose, P. 2011. Acute infective conjunctivitis in primary care: Who needs antibiotics? An individual patient data meta-analysis. *Br J Gen Pract*; 61(590):e542–e548.

Public Health England. 2017. Guidance on infection control in schools and other child care settings. www.publichealth.hscni.net/publications/guidance-infection-control-schools-and-other-childcare-settings-0.

RCGP. 2016. Thousands of GP appointments 'lost' due to children with conjunctivitis being turned away from nursery, says RCGP. www.rcgp.org.uk/news/2016/november/thousands-of-gp-appointments-lost-due-to-children-with-conjunctivitis-being-turned-away-from-nursery.aspx.

Sheikh, A., Hurwitz, B., van Schayck, C.P., McLean, S., and Nurmatov, U. 2012. Antibiotics versus placebo for acute bacterial conjunctivitis. *Cochrane Database Syst Rev*; (9). Art. No.: CD001211. doi: 10.1002/14651858.CD001211.pub3.

BLEPHARITIS

Inflammation of the eyelids with stickiness and characteristic yellow scales at roots of eyelashes. May occur alongside conjunctivitis or on its own. Seborrhoeic dermatitis may co-exist.

- Remove scales by applying warm compresses, then wiping lids twice daily for 2 weeks with cotton wool dipped in diluted baby shampoo, or a pinch of sodium bicarbonate in a cup of cooled, boiled water. Long-term lid hygiene should be recommended
- Patients with blepharitis often also have dry eyes
- Chloramphenicol[PB] eye ointment may be added if lid hygiene alone is ineffective
- Severe and persistent symptoms may require oral antibiotics

Reference

Lindsley, K., Matsumura, S., Hatef, E., and Akpek, E.K. 2012. Interventions for chronic blepharitis. *Cochrane Database Syst Rev*; (5). Art. No.: CD005556. doi: 10.1002/14651858.CD005556.pub2.

ALLERGIC CONJUNCTIVITIS

- Bilateral itchy eyes
- Generalised conjunctival inflammation
- Recurrent symptoms
- Sneezing, itchy throat
- History of triggers, for example, animal fur, hay fever
- Watering rather than discharge

Self-care
- Avoid triggers, if possible
- Oral antihistamine (e.g. loratadine or cetirizine)
- An antihistamine eyedrop is available OTC (Otrivine-Antistin®[PBC]), but this also contains a vasoconstrictor, so should not be used for more than 3 days
- Sodium cromoglicate eye drops are an alternative but are slower acting. They may sting

Action
- If self-care is ineffective, prescribe azelastine[PBC] eyedrops (or sodium cromoglicate eyedrops if patient is pregnant or breastfeeding)

Reference

Castillo, M., Scott, N.W., Mustafa, M.Z., Mustafa, M.S., and Azuara-Blanco, A. 2015. Topical antihistamines and mast cell stabilisers for treating seasonal and perennial allergic conjunctivitis. *Cochrane Database Syst Rev*; (6). Art. No.: CD009566. doi: 10.1002/14651858.CD009566.pub2.

DRY EYES

Older patients are more commonly affected, eyes feel gritty but look normal, and vision unaffected. Blepharitis is often also present.

- Be aware that dry eyes can cause patients to experience symptoms of watery eyes – the excess tears, however, are not oily enough to be effective
- Reduce the use of contact lenses
- Stop medication that may exacerbate dry eyes, for example, antihistamines
- Avoid long periods without blinking (e.g. staring at a computer or gaming screen)
- Artificial tears help but must be used frequently (hypromellose or Viscotears®, available OTC)
- Omega-3 supplements may be useful

References

American Academy of Ophthalmology. 2013. Dry eye syndrome PPP. www.aao.org/preferred-practice-pattern/dry-eye-syndrome-ppp--2013.

Epitropoulos, A.T., Donnenfeld, E.D., Shah, Z.A., Holland, E.J., Gross, M., Faulkner, W.J., Matossian, C. et al. Effect of oral re-esterified omega-3 nutritional supplementation on dry eyes. *Cornea*; 35(9):1185–1191.

STYE

A staphylococcal infection of one eyelash root causing an acute painful swelling on lash margin (swelling deeper in the lid would indicate a chalazion (see below)). May have a small area of pus at the tip.

Self-care

- Warm compresses three to four times daily
- Advise about risk of infecting others, use own face cloth and towel
- Avoid using makeup and contact lenses
- Advise the patient not to puncture the stye themselves
- Topical antibiotics are not recommended

Reference

NICE CKS. 2015. Styes (hordeola). https://cks.nice.org.uk/styes-hordeola#!scenario.

CHALAZION (MEIBOMIAN CYST)

This is a firm, localised swelling in one eyelid (not on the lash margin) developing over several weeks. It is initially uncomfortable and is caused by blockage in drainage of an eyelid gland, not an infection.

Self-care

- Warm compresses three to four times daily to liquefy cyst contents
- Massage cyst in direction of eyelashes twice daily using clean fingers or cotton buds
- Clean eyelid margin with cotton bud dipped in baby shampoo diluted 1:10 with warm water
- Usually resolve within 6–8 weeks
- Antibiotic therapy is not recommended unless cellulitis is suspected
- If not resolving, then ophthalmology outpatient referral for surgery may be needed, particularly if pulling eyelid away from the eye or causing excessive watering

References

Carlisle, R.T., and Digiovanni, J. 2015. Differential diagnosis of the swollen red eyelid. *Am Fam Physician*; 92(2). www.aafp.org/afp/2015/0715/p106.pdf.

NICE CKS. 2015. Meibomian cyst (chalazion). https://cks.nice.org.uk/meibomian-cyst-chalazion.

SUBCONJUNCTIVAL HAEMORRHAGE

This may sometimes be confused with conjunctivitis. It causes a sudden uniform red area in the eye with a sharp edge. You should be able to see the posterior margin. There is no discomfort, discharge or deterioration in vision. It is usually caused by minor trauma but sometimes may be the first presenting symptom of hypertension. Lubricant drops such as hypromellose or Viscotears® may help to ease any discomfort.

- Since it is asymptomatic, the patient may have detected it after looking in the mirror or someone else alerting them
- Reassurance is usually all that is needed
- Check blood pressure and examine the margins of the red area
- 🚩 After trauma, if the posterior margin of the haemorrhage is not visible, this should raise suspicion of a fracture of the orbital bone or an intracranial haemorrhage
- 🚩 If taking warfarin, check international normalised ratio (INR)

Reference

Patient.info. 2017. Subconjunctival haemorrhage. https://patient.info/doctor/subconjunctival-haemorrhage-pro.

CORNEAL ULCER

Caused by a viral infection, for example, herpes simplex or varicella zoster.

- 🚩 History: pain, photophobia, unilateral symptoms, no discharge, reduced visual acuity
- Examination: unilateral red eye. Cornea may be hazy with red edge
- Test: stain with fluorescein and observe with light (ideally blue light) and magnification. Ulcer stains green
- Action: same-day referral to Ophthalmology (slit lamp examination is needed to confirm the diagnosis)

Reference

NICE CKS. 2016. Red eye. https://cks.nice.org.uk/red-eye.

CHAPTER 7

Neurology

HEADACHE

Headache is common, but patients often fear that they have an underlying brain tumour. Fortunately, this is rare, being the cause of only 1 in 600 people presenting in primary care with new onset of headaches. Severe headaches are not necessarily the ones of greater concern. Typical features that are either reassuring or suspicious are given in Table 7.1. Many common infections cause headache (leading to concerns about meningitis), but overall, the commonest cause of headache is psychosocial stress.

History

- We all get headaches – what is different about this one?
- What is worrying you? (often a brain tumour)
- Duration: episodic/unremitting
- Onset: sudden/gradual
- Aura? (visual or other)
- Timing: waking from sleep/later in the day/related to menstrual cycle
- Severity of pain
- Quality: sharp/like a pressure or band/throbbing
- Site
- Any known triggers?
- Exacerbating factors, for example, coughing or change in posture
- Relieving factors, for example, rest or darkness
- Impact on daily life
- Treatments tried and how often
- Previous recurrent headaches
- Family history of similar headaches
- Depression/anxiety/insomnia
- Sleep pattern/shift work
- Fluid, alcohol, and caffeine intake
- Recent new medication (e.g. nitrates/calcium channel blockers)
- Oestrogen-containing contraceptives
- Associated symptoms (ask whether simultaneous or before headache):
  - Visual disturbance/eye pain
  - Nausea/vomiting
  - Any feverish illness and its symptoms
  - Sinus problems
  - Neck pain
  - 🚩 Rash
  - 🚩 Scalp or temple tenderness
  - 🚩 Neurological symptoms, for example, sensory disturbance, double vision, incoordination
- 🚩 Recent head injury
- 🚩 Cancer (including past history) or human immunodeficiency virus (HIV)
- 🚩 Carbon monoxide exposure
- 🚩 Pregnancy (see Box 7.2)

Table 7.1 Features of headache

Reassuring	Suspicious
On the top of my head	Always there when I wake up
Like a band around my head	Wakes me from sleep
It can last all day	Localised
It can come on at any time	Sudden onset
I have had it for years on and off	Hurts more when I cough or bend over
Family history of similar headaches	Associated with neurological or visual symptoms

Examination

- Temperature (if infection suspected)
- Blood pressure (this must be really high – usually above 180/110 mmHg – to cause headache, but also it is important to check because migraine is associated with hypertension)
- Heart rate (while infection would drive tachycardia, space-occupying lesions or intracranial hypertension may cause a reflex slowing of the heart rate)
- Palpate temporal arteries for tenderness, particularly if patient over 50 years
- Check for neck or back stiffness, if meningitis or cerebral haemorrhage is suspected

Tests

- Erythrocyte sedimentation rate (ESR) if giant cell (temporal) arteritis suspected (Box 7.1)

Self-care

- Reassure (if appropriate) that headache without neurological or visual symptoms is very unlikely to indicate brain tumour
- Regular meals, adequate fluids, avoid sudden changes in caffeine consumption
- Stress reduction or management (e.g. exercise, meditation, relaxation techniques. Apps such as Breathe2Relax or Headspace may be helpful)
- Simple analgesics for occasional use, for example, ibuprofen[P] (most people have only tried paracetamol)
- Analgesics for headache should not be taken on more than 10 days per month
- Avoid codeine (high risk of withdrawal headache)
- Adequate, but not excessive, time for sleep
- A headache diary may be useful
- If headaches are persistent, consider acupuncture and arrange assessment by General Practitioner (GP)

BOX 7.1 GIANT CELL (TEMPORAL) ARTERITIS

This autoimmune condition causes inflammation in small- to medium-sized arteries, especially those on the temples. It is more common over the age of 50, but occasionally it may affect younger people. The headache is severe, usually unilateral and often associated with tenderness of the scalp and temples, aching of the jaw muscles on eating and visual disturbance. There may be fever and fatigue; 40% also have associated weakness of other muscles with morning stiffness, aches and weight loss (polymyalgia rheumatica). It is a 'red flag' because it may cause sudden occlusion of important blood vessels, resulting in blindness, stroke or myocardial infarction, so patients in whom it is suspected should be referred urgently to a doctor. The patient should start prednisolone[I] without waiting for test results (initial dose 60 mg with visual symptoms, 40–60 mg without (minimum 0.75 mg/kg)), plus aspirin[PBCI] 75 mg/day and omeprazole[Q] 20 mg/day. Referral is needed for temporal artery biopsy or specialist colour duplex ultrasound (which should be performed within 2 weeks of starting prednisolone), and a raised ESR will help in confirming the diagnosis. If the diagnosis is suspected and the ESR is not very high, check the CRP and continue the treatment until the patient is seen by a specialist. Once the diagnosis is confirmed histologically, long-term treatment is needed with prednisolone.

Reference

Ninan, J., Lester, S., and Hill, C. 2016. Giant cell arteritis. *Best Pract Res Clin Rheumatol*; 30(1):169–188.

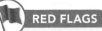 **RED FLAGS**

- Previous cancer (*possible cerebral metastases; refer to GP or Oncology*)
- Pregnant and blood pressure >140/90 (*pre-eclampsia, Box 7.2; refer to Obstetrics*)
- New-onset headaches over age 50 (*needs investigation; refer to GP*)
- First episode of migraine over age 40 (*needs investigation; refer to GP*)
- First migraine/focal migraine in woman taking oestrogen–containing contraceptive (*risk of stroke, change contraceptive method to non-hormonal or progesterone-only*)
- Sudden 'thunderclap' headache (*possible subarachnoid haemorrhage; call 999*)
- Recent head injury (*possible subdural haemorrhage; refer Surgical same-day*)
- Other symptoms suggesting meningitis (*call 999 and give benzylpenicillin*)
- Suspected carbon monoxide poisoning (*refer same-day to Medical if currently symptomatic; otherwise check appliances. Gas Emergency Helpline: 0800 111 999*)
- Eye pain (*consider acute glaucoma; refer to urgent Eye Clinic if suspected*)
- Headache waking from sleep (*possible cerebral tumour or cluster headache; refer to GP*)
- Neurological symptoms (*possible cerebral haemorrhage/tumour; refer to GP*)
- Temporal artery tenderness (*possible giant cell arteritis; measure ESR, start steroids and refer urgently to GP/Rheumatology/Ophthalmology*)
- Worsening/persistent headaches (*need investigation; refer to GP*)

BOX 7.2 PRE-ECLAMPSIA

- Defined as new hypertension after 20 weeks' gestation with significant proteinuria
- More common in the second half of first pregnancy, first pregnancy with a new partner or in subsequent pregnancies after previous episodes
- Symptoms may include:
  - Severe increasing headaches
  - Visual problems, for example, blurred vision, flashing lights, double vision
  - Pain in epigastrium or right upper quadrant
  - Vomiting
  - Breathlessness
  - Sudden swelling of face, hands or feet

Refer to Obstetrics urgently if:

- New hypertension (BP > 140/90) and:
  - Symptoms of pre-eclampsia *or*
  - BP 160/110 or higher *or*
  - Urine dip positive for 1+ or more protein
- No hypertension but proteinuria on dipstick and symptoms of pre-clampsia

Seek urgent specialist advice for all other women with symptoms of pre-clampsia *or* new hypertension *or* proteinuria

Reference

NICE CKS. 2015. Hypertension in pregnancy. cks.nice.org.uk/hypertension-in-pregnancy.

Note: there is no point in referring a patient presenting with headache and no eye symptoms to an optician, unless you feel that this would reduce their anxiety about a tumour. Poor vision is most unlikely to be the sole cause of headache, and if you are concerned enough to feel that the patient needs examination of the optic disc for signs of raised intracranial pressure, then urgent referral to a doctor is needed.

References

Kernick, D., Stapley, S., Goadsby, P.J., and Hamilton, W.W. 2008. What happens to new-onset headache presented to primary care? A case–cohort study using electronic primary care records. *Cephalalgia*; 28:1188–1195.

MacGregor, E.A., Steiner, T.J., and Davies, P.T.G. 2010. Guidelines for all healthcare professionals in the diagnosis and management of migraine, tension-type, cluster and medication-overuse headache. *British Association for the Study of Headache.* www.bash.org.uk/wp-content/uploads/2012/07/10102-BASH-Guidelines-update-2_v5-1-indd.pdf.

NICE CG 150. 2012. Headaches in over 12s: Diagnosis and management. www.nice.org.uk/guidance/cg150/chapter/Update-information.

NICE CKS. 2013. Headache – assessment. cks.nice.org.uk/headache-assessment.

MIGRAINE

Migraine affects 12% of adults and 10% of children and is commoner in females. At least 90% of people with migraine experience a first attack before the age of 40. Symptoms of the aura do not last more than 60 minutes (typically 20–30 minutes) and resolve before the pain begins. Early symptoms such as emotional or personality changes, muddled thinking, excessive tiredness, yawning, pallor, visual disturbances and restlessness may start 1–48 hours before the headache. A close relative or a friend may notice these changes before the patient does. In children, visual symptoms are less common and may be simultaneous with the headache, or they may have abdominal pain, vomiting or dizziness without headache.

Migraine causes instability in the size of the blood vessels in the head and the neck, although the initial event that starts an attack occurs in the brainstem. It is helpful for patients to be informed that the reason they are susceptible to migraine, resulting from triggers that do not cause headache in other people, is down to an inherited predisposition. There is usually a family history of migraine, more often on the mother's side.

A wide variety of factors are known to trigger migraine:

- Change in stress level
- Excessive sensory stimuli, for example, bright light, noise
- Premenstrual hormone changes
- Missing meals
- Overexertion
- Sleep disturbance – too much or too little
- Change in climate
- Hypoxia

Dietary factors are often suspected but rarely found; searching too hard may divert attention away from more likely factors, such as those mentioned previously. The widespread belief that chocolate is a trigger lacks evidence (Lippi et al., 2014). It is more likely to be a food craving in the prodromal phase. Alcohol does not cause migraine initially but can trigger an attack as its effects wear off. For most people, the attacks seem to be multifactorial, and it is often not possible to identify any one trigger which always causes migraine or, when avoided, stops all attacks. Often there is a buildup of different triggers, with a 'last straw' tipping the sufferer over the threshold and resulting in a migraine. Whatever the cause, the final part of the sequence of events leading to symptoms involves the neurotransmitter 5-hydroxytryptamine (serotonin, 5-HT).

Migraine associated with difficulty in reading, particularly in children or young people, may respond to colour tinting of spectacles. Referral to an optometrist for an intuitive colorimeter test may both help the migraine and (importantly) improve educational potential (Evans et al., 2016). Adults with frequent dyspepsia or heartburn as well as migraine should be tested for *Helicobacter pylori* – if the presence of Helicobacter is confirmed, eradication therapy may abolish the migraine as well as the gut symptoms (Su et al., 2014).

Diagnostic history of migraine

- Episodes lasting 4–72 hours
- Often unilateral (though not always)
- Pulsating/throbbing
- Moderate or severe pain
- Exacerbated by physical activity
- Nausea and/or vomiting
- Photophobia or phonophobia (sensitivity to noise)
- Focal migraine may also cause one of the following types of aura:
  - Visual symptoms (e.g. flickering lights and/or partial visual loss)

- Sensory symptoms (pins and needles and/or numbness)
- Dysphasia (speech disturbance)

Self-care

- Simple analgesics (paracetamol, aspirin[PBCI], or ibuprofen[P]) work for many sufferers, but must be taken early in the attack
- If there is associated nausea, it is important to treat this as well, with an antiemetic such as buccal prochlorperazine[PBCQ] (OTC – see section that follows for further information), ideally taken at the first sign of symptoms
- If simple analgesics are ineffective, consider sumatriptan[CQ] (adult dose 50 mg. If the migraine improves but recurs, a second dose of 50 mg can be taken after at least 2 hours if required. Packs of two 50 mg tablets OTC)
- The Migraine Trust is a research charity providing helpful information for patients (www.migrainetrust.org)

Advice

- If taking combined oral contraceptive (COC) or other oestrogen-containing contraceptive and first episode of migraine, or migraine with aura/focal symptoms, advise stopping COC immediately and discuss alternative contraceptive methods

Prescription

For migraine in adults, NICE recommends a combination of a triptan and a non-steroidal anti-inflammatory drug (NSAID), although monotherapy with a triptan is nearly as effective. Naratriptan[PBCQ] is our first-choice triptan because of its low side effect profile and low rate of migraine recurrence. If it is effective for the patient, they can continue to use it without a high burden of side effects; if it is not effective, other triptans are available that have greater efficacy. People vary in their response, so if the initial treatment is not working well, it is worth trying an alternative triptan or NSAID (Belvis et al., 2009; Saper et al., 2001). Avoid enteric-coated NSAIDs as they may be too slow in onset to be effective. An anti-emetic can increase the effectiveness of the analgesic as well as reducing nausea; prochlorperazine[PBCQ] is available in a buccal tablet and, therefore, does not require the patient to 'keep it down'. If nausea and vomiting are prominent, then an alternative route of analgesia may be needed, for example, diclofenac[PC] suppositories or zolmitriptan[PBCQ] nasal spray.

Doses for adults

- Naratriptan[PBCQ] 2.5 mg. If the migraine improves but recurs, a second dose of 2.5 mg can be taken after at least 4 hours if required. Maximum 5 mg/24 hours
- Buccal prochlorperazine[PBCQ] (OTC) 3–6 mg up to twice daily; tablets to be placed high between upper lip and gum and left to dissolve
- Diclofenac[PC] 100 mg suppository once in 24 hours
- Zolmitriptan[PBCQ] nasal spray 5 mg as soon as possible after onset into one nostril only. If the migraine improves but recurs, a second dose of 5 mg can be taken after at least 2 hours if required. Maximum 10 mg/24 hr

 RED FLAGS

- Migraine lasting more than 72 hours and not responding to usual care (*status migrainosus; refer same-day to Medical for parenteral treatment*)
- First episode of migraine over the age of 40 (*needs investigation; refer to GP*)
- First migraine/focal migraine in woman taking oestrogen–containing contraceptive (*risk of stroke; change contraceptive method to nonhormonal or progesterone-only*)

References

Belvis, R., Pagonabarraga, J., and Kulisevsky, J. 2009. Individual triptan selection in migraine attack therapy. *Recent Pat CNS Drug Discov*; 4(1):70–81. http://ukpmc.ac.uk/abstract/MED/19149716.

Evans, B.J., and Allen, P.M. 2016. A systematic review of controlled trials on visual stress using intuitive overlays or the intuitive colorimeter. *J Optom*; 9(4):205–218.

Evans, E.W., and Lorber, K.C. 2008. Use of 5-HT1 agonists in pregnancy. *Ann Pharmacother*; 42(4):543–549. http://ukpmc.ac.uk/abstract/MED/18349309.

Law, S., Derry, S., and Moore, R.A. 2016. Sumatriptan plus naproxen for the treatment of acute migraine attacks in adults. *Cochrane Database Syst Rev*; (4). Art. No.: CD008541. doi: 10.1002/14651858.CD008541.pub3.

Linde, K., Allais, G., Brinkhaus, B., Fei, Y., Mehring, M., Vertosick, E.A., Vickers, A., and White, A.R. 2016. Acupuncture for the prevention of episodic migraine. *Cochrane Database Syst Rev*; (6). Art. No.: CD001218. doi: 10.1002/14651858.CD001218.pub3.

Lippi, G., Mattiuzzi, C., and Cervellin, G. 2014. Chocolate and migraine: The history of an ambiguous association. *Acta Bio-medica*; 85(3):216–221.

National Migraine Centre. 2017. Migraine triggers. www.nationalmigrainecentre.org.uk/migraine-and-headaches/migraine-and-headache-factsheets/migraine-triggers/.

NICE CKS. 2016. Migraine. https://cks.nice.org.uk/migraine.

Pringsheim, T., and Becker, W.J. 2014. Triptans for symptomatic treatment of migraine headache. *BMJ*; 348:g2285. www.bmj.com/content/348/bmj.g2285.abstract. doi: 10.1136/bmj.g2285.

Saper, J.R. 2001. What matters is not the differences between triptans, but the differences between patients. *Arch Neurol*; 58(9):1481–1482.

Su, J., Zhou, X., and Zhang, G. 2014. Association between Helicobacter pylori infection and migraine: A meta-analysis. *World J Gastroenterol*; 20(40):14965–14972.

Utku, U., Gokce, M., Benli, E.M., Dinc, A., and Tuncel, D. 2014. Intra-venous chlorpromazine with fluid treatment in status migrainosus. *Clin Neurol Neurosurg*; 119:4–5. doi: 10.1016/j.clineuro.2014.01.002.

DIZZINESS

There are fundamentally two types of dizziness: vertigo (caused by a disturbance of the balance system) and fainting/near-fainting (caused by a lack of oxygen in the brain).

History

- What is worrying you? (often a stroke)
- Duration
- Circumstances:
  - If triggered or exacerbated by movement, suggests vertigo
  - If occurring at rest or sitting/lying still, suggests epileptic cause
  - If triggered by exercise, suggests a cardiac cause
  - If triggered by heat, emotion, or toiletting, suggests a vasovagal cause (simple faint)
- If loss of consciousness, try to obtain written eyewitness account. Was there any injury or incontinence?
- Nature (when you have dizzy spells, do you feel the world spin around you as if you had just got off a playground roundabout?):
  - Spinning or movement (vertigo – see Box 7.3)
  - Faint feeling (as if about to black out)
- Previous episodes/ear surgery
- Recent head injury
- Recent blood loss
- Pregnancy
- Heart disease
- Diabetes
- Medication (especially if newly started or increased, for example, antihypertensives, antidiabetic medicines, tramadol, gabapentin, antidepressants)
- Associated symptoms:
  - Nausea
  - Earache
  - Viral infection

- Sudden deafness/tinnitus
- Headache/photophobia/visual loss/clumsiness/other neurological symptoms
- Palpitations
- Chest pain
- Family history of sudden adult death

Examination

- If vertigo, check ears and look for nystagmus on lateral gaze (suggests vestibular neuronitis)
- Blood pressure, sitting and standing (wait 2 minutes)
- Pulse rate and rhythm
- Pallor/anaemia

Tests

- Full blood count (FBC) if anaemia is suspected
- Capillary blood glucose if hypoglycaemia is suspected
- Electrocardiogram (ECG) if cardiac cause is suspected (but a normal ECG does not exclude a cardiac cause)

VERTIGO

Vestibular neuronitis (or labyrinthitis), benign paroxysmal positional vertigo (BPPV), and vestibular migraine are common causes of vertigo in primary care (see Box 7.3). Other diagnoses are possible, for example, Ménière's disease and cerebral ischaemia. It is worth checking the ears for signs of infection. Nystagmus may also be seen, especially on lateral gaze.

Self-care

- Dizziness is common, and nausea often accompanies it
- Symptoms usually settle but may sometimes take several weeks
- Encourage activity, even if it worsens the vertigo, as it can speed recovery
- Driving or other critical tasks may be affected (see DVLA form DIZ1)
- Consider taking buccal prochlorperazine[PBCQ] (OTC) or cinnarizine[PBC] (OTC) for no more than 10 days. These are for symptomatic relief, not a cure; they cause sedation (and may delay recovery)
- For BPPV, simple Brandt–Daroff exercises also may be helpful (see Sandwell and West Birmingham Hospitals, 2012)

BOX 7.3 VERTIGO

Vertigo: Common differential diagnoses

	Vestibular neuronitis	BPPV	Vestibular migraine	Cerebral ischaemia
Background	Recent URTI	Spontaneous, or after head trauma	Migraine history, or family history	History of cardiovascular disease
Characteristic signs/symptoms	Nystagmus	Brought on by movement	Other migraine symptoms, maybe no headache	Other neurological symptoms
Associated features	Nausea and vomiting	Vertigo lasts less than a minute	Vertigo lasts 5 minutes to 72 hours	Maybe visual disturbance, drowsiness or headache
Timing	One episode may give symptoms over 18 months	Recurrent	Recurrent	Usually single event

Doses for adults

- Buccal prochlorperazine[PBCQ] (OTC) 3–6 mg up to twice daily; tablets to be placed high between upper lip and gum and left to dissolve
- Cinnarizine [PBC] (OTC) 30 mg three times daily

RED FLAGS

- Neurological symptoms or signs (*suspect cerebrovascular disease/stroke; convey via 999 if suspected acute stroke, otherwise refer to Medical*)
- Headache/photophobia/new tinnitus (*suspect brain or ear disease; refer to Medical or ENT outpatients*)
- Sudden unilateral hearing loss (*possible vascular or immune disease of cochlea; refer to ENT urgently*)
- Head injury in previous 3 weeks, especially if on anticoagulant (*possible subdural haemorrhage; refer to Surgical same-day*)
- Previous ear surgery (*refer to ENT outpatients*)
- Vertigo not improving after 1 week or not resolved after 6 weeks (*possible BPPV, acoustic neuroma, cerebrovascular disease; refer to ENT outpatients*)

References

International Headache Society. 2016. Vestibular migraine. www.ichd-3.org/appendix/a1-migraine/a1-6-episodic-synd romes-that-may-be-associated-with-migraine/a1-6-6-vestibular-migraine/.

Newson, L. 2014. Dizziness, giddiness, and feeling faint. Patient.info. patient.info/doctor/dizziness-giddiness-and-feeling-faint.

NICE CKS. 2011. Vestibular neuronitis. cks.nice.org.uk/vestibular-neuronitis.

Sandwell and West Birmingham Hospitals. 2012. Brandt-Daroff exercises. www.swbh.nhs.uk/wp-content/uploads/2012/07/Brandt-Daroff-Exercises-ML3094.pdf.

FAINTING

Fainting occurs when there is not enough oxygen available to the brain. Check the capillary blood glucose to exclude hypoglycaemia and a full blood count to exclude anaemia. Vasovagal syncope, hypotension, hypovolaemia, anaemia, arrhythmias, cardiac failure and epilepsy are among the many causes of feeling faint (see Box 7.4).

BOX 7.4 FEELING FAINT

Feeling faint: Common differential diagnoses (NB many other causes are possible)

	Vasovagal	Hypotensive	Cardiac	Epileptic
Background	Any age, but first episode usually under 40 years	History of blood loss, diarrhoea, or vomiting	Commoner in elderly	Any age
Typical trigger	Situational trigger, for example, blood test, prolonged standing, micturition	Symptoms exacerbated by standing	During exercise or when lying down	May occur in a situation unusual for other causes – like sitting at rest
Features/ associations	Loss of consciousness not usually more than 20 seconds	Maybe a low fluid intake	Preceding nausea or sweating	Aura before, or drowsiness/amnesia after
Features/ associations	Pallor and sweating	On antihypertensive medicines	Palpitation, dyspnoea or chest pain	Twitching, jerking or abnormal movements
Features/ associations	Most common cause – often preceded by feeling faint and vision narrowing	BP low or drops >20/10 mmHg within 3 minutes of standing	Known cardiac disease or abnormal ECG	Injury or lateral tongue biting

Self-care

- Avoid hot baths and prolonged standing, especially in the heat
- Drink adequate fluids; have two large glasses of water before situations that are likely to make you faint
- When getting out of bed, roll over and sit on the edge of the bed for a few minutes before standing
- Avoid your own triggers and be aware of your warning signs
- At the first sign of feeling faint, lie down flat with your legs up on a chair or against a wall or sit down with your head between your knees
- If this is not possible, squat down on your heels. Both positions move blood from the legs back into the circulation
- When you feel better, get up slowly, but return to the position if symptoms return

RED FLAGS

- Family history of sudden adult death (*high risk of fatal arrhythmia; refer to Cardiology urgently*)
- Systolic BP < 90 mmHg or drops by more than 20 mmHg on standing (*suspect medication or other causes of postural hypotension; refer to GP or Medical*)
- Sustained increase in heart rate by ≥ 30 beats/min within 10 min of standing (*suspect postural tachycardia syndrome; refer to GP or Medical*)
- Heart disease, known or suspected because of palpitations or chest pain (*refer to GP or Medical*)
- Injury or lateral tongue biting during episode (*suggests epilepsy; refer to Neurology*)

References

Payne, J. 2015. Syncope. Patient.info. patient.info/doctor/syncope.

Quinn, J.V., Stiell, I.G., McDermott, D.A., Sellers, K.L., Kohn, M.A., and Wells, G.A. 2004. Derivation of the San Francisco syncope rule to predict patients with short-term serious outcomes. *Ann Emerg Med*; 43(2):224–232.

CHAPTER 8

Skin

INTRODUCTION

Healthcare professionals often find skin problems daunting at first. Remember two important principles, which apply equally to all types of minor illness:

- **Find out and address the patient's agenda.** This is commonly:
  - (For a rash) is it meningitis?
  - Is it contagious?
  - (For an isolated lesion) is it cancer?
- **Take a good history.** This is where to find the diagnosis – your examination is for confirmation. The four most useful questions are about:
  - Fever/malaise
  - Distribution
  - Itch or pain
  - Duration
- Other questions:
  - Are the spots of different ages? Are they spreading?
  - Any previous episodes?
  - Have any suspected triggers been identified?
  - Are there any associated symptoms?
  - Anyone else affected?

The Primary Care Dermatology Society (PCDS, www.pcds.org.uk) has a useful website with diagnostic algorithms as well as management advice. It may be helpful to compare the patient's rash with photos; Dermnet (www.dermnetnz.org) or Dermis (www.dermis.net) are good online resources, or use one of the many books available.

It is quite likely that you may not be able to make a definite diagnosis. If you have addressed the patient's concerns and ruled out serious illness, this may not matter. If the problem does not resolve, the patient should make an appointment with a doctor.

Reference

Ashton, R., Leppard, B., and Cooper, H. 2014. Differential Diagnosis in Dermatology, 4th edition. CRC Press, London. ISBN-13:978-1909368729. *This book has very useful algorithms that explain the likely diagnoses for a particular presentation and their distinguishing features.*

RASHES

History
- Duration
- Unwell with fever/malaise
- Distribution
- Itch or pain
- Did all spots appear at same time or sequentially?
- Is rash constant, spreading, or coming and going?
- Previous episodes
- Any contacts who are itching
- Any new medication

- Any identified triggers
- What has been tried already and what was the response?

Examination

- Distribution/symmetry across the midline
- Discrete (separate 'spots') or confluent (merging 'rash')
- Colour, but beware: in darkly pigmented skin it is difficult to assess the degree of inflammation
- Does the rash blanch on pressure?
- Surface – feel with fingertips
- Are the areas:
  - Wheal-like (irregular, raised, blotchy)
  - Flat (macules) or raised (papules)
  - Containing fluid (vesicles or pustules)
- For itchy rashes, are burrows visible on the hands?
- If patient unwell, check:
  - Temperature
  - Pulse rate
  - Respiratory rate
  - Capillary refill time in children
  - Blood pressure in adults

Tests

- A swab for bacterial culture may be helpful in cellulitis or infected eczema
- Skin scrapings or 'dust' from around the edges of the nail may be sent for fungal culture – the results may take around 3 weeks. Do not refrigerate the sample

Now see the different sections:

A. Acute generalised itchy rash

B. Rash in a seriously ill patient

C. Rash in a febrile patient

D. Purple rashes

E. Localised rashes

F. Localised bacterial infections

G. Miscellaneous

ACUTE GENERALISED ITCHY RASH

1. Chickenpox
2. Urticaria
3. Scabies
4. Pityriasis rosea
5. Eczema (see section on Miscellaneous)

CHICKENPOX

- Caused by the varicella zoster virus (also called herpes zoster)
- Incubation period 10–21 days. Most infectious in the 48 hours before spots appear
- Significant exposure is regarded as over 5 minutes face-to-face or 15 minutes in same room
- May cause fever, headache, and malaise (tends to be more marked in adults)
- Separate itchy papules at different stages of development, turning to vesicles

Self-care

- Crotamiton^{PB} lotion OTC (keep in fridge, avoid application to nipple area if breastfeeding) may be used to reduce itching. Cooling gels are popular, although there is little evidence to support their use. Calamine has a drying effect and is no longer recommended
- Chlorphenamine^{PBI} is useful at night because of its sedative action, but sedation may be unacceptable (4 mg at bedtime, repeated after 4 hours if necessary, for adults)
- Non-sedating antihistamines are probably ineffective
- Avoid ibuprofen as it increases the risk of secondary bacterial infection
- Porridge oats in fine mesh (e.g. tights) held under running bath water may be soothing
- Infectious until all lesions have crusted over (usually five days). Avoid contact with vulnerable people (see below)

Action

For people with the infection:

- Prescribe aciclovir to the immunosuppressed (800 mg five times a day for 7 days for adults)
- Prescribe aciclovir if onset of rash <24 hours ago and any of the following:
    - >14 years of age
    - Severe pain
    - Dense or oral rash
    - Smoker
- Chickenpox is a notifiable disease in Northern Ireland

For contacts of people with the infection:

- Consider varicella zoster immunoglobulin (VZIG) for any of the following:
    - Pregnant; if VZIG is in short supply, aciclovir may be prescribed to pregnant women >20 weeks' gestation instead (Public Health England, 2018)
    - Immunosuppressed
    - Neonates ≤7 days of age
    - Infants <1 year of age who were born prematurely, under 1 kg birth weight or with significant co-morbidity

This may need to be organised through your local Health Protection Team. See Public Health England (2017) guidance on immunoglobulin.

RED FLAGS

- Immunosuppressed (*give aciclovir; seek specialist advice*)
- Pregnant/less than 4 weeks after childbirth (*seek specialist advice*)
- Baby aged under 4 weeks (30% mortality) (*may need IV aciclovir; seek specialist advice*)
- Breathless/confused/severe headache/petechial rash (*pneumonia, encephalitis and thrombocytopenia are possible complications of chickenpox; pregnant women are at highest risk. Admit urgently under Medical/Paediatrics*)
- **Suspected secondary bacterial infection** (risk increased if the patient is treated with oral corticosteroid or an NSAID such as ibuprofen). Some lesions become painful rather than itchy, and may weep purulent fluid; a second phase of fever develops (*consider admission to hospital if any sign of sepsis. If treating in primary care, take a swab from any weeping lesion for bacterial culture, and prescribe both flucloxacillin and amoxicillin. This combination should cover common skin pathogens such as Staphylococcus and Streptococcus, which has been implicated in life-threatening secondary infections*)

References

NICE CKS. 2016. Chickenpox. cks.nice.org.uk/chickenpox.

Public Health England. 2016. Guidance on viral rash in pregnancy. www.gov.uk/government/publications/viral-rash-in-pregnancy.

Public Health England. 2017. Immunoglobulin: when to use. www.gov.uk/government/publications/immunoglobulin-when-to-use.

Public Health England. 2018. Use of Varicella Zoster Immunoglobulin in pregnancy during supply shortage: advice to GPs, obstetricians and midwives. https://assets.publishing.service.gov.uk/government/uploads/system/uploads/attachment_data/file/724859/PHE_VZIG_interim_guidance_for_GPs_obstetricians_and_midwives.pdf

UK Medicines Information. 2016. Do NSAIDs increase the risk of severe skin reactions in children with chickenpox? www.sps.nhs.uk/articles/do-nsaids-increase-the-risk-of-severe-skin-reactions-in-children-with-chickenpox/.

URTICARIA

This is a rash triggered by the immune system either appropriately (infection), inappropriately (allergy) or for an unknown reason (idiopathic). It is caused by dilation of capillaries and the release of histamine from mast cells, causing leakage of plasma into the skin.

- Also called 'nettle rash' (the botanical name of the nettle is *Urtica*) or 'hives'
- Usually an itchy rash that comes and goes over a few hours
- Raised paler wheals on a background flare
- Accompanied by burning or itching
- Common causes include:
  - Drugs (e.g. aspirin, penicillins, NSAIDs, ACE inhibitors)
  - Viral infection
  - Food allergy (e.g. nuts, strawberries)
  - Gastrointestinal upset (associated with *H. pylori*)
  - Bites and stings
  - Heat or cold (e.g. 'prickly heat')
  - Vigorous exercise
  - Pressure
  - Psychosocial stress ('stress rash')
- 🚩 Check for angio-oedema – tongue and lip swelling/wheeze/hypotension
- 🚩 If wheals last more than 24 hours and leave a mark, possible underlying vasculitis
- 🚩 If unexplained joint pains, could have underlying autoimmune cause
- 🚩 Urticaria in children with food allergy triggers can herald future anaphylaxis

Self-care

- Oral (not topical) antihistamines: loratadine or cetirizine (10 mg once daily for adults)
- Chlorphenamine[PBI] may be added if sedation desirable/acceptable (4 mg every 4–6 hours; maximum 24 mg per day for adults)
- Avoid any identified triggers

Prescription

- If the above is ineffective, consider changing to fexofenadine[PC] (120 mg once daily for adults)
- Allergy specialists may recommend increasing the dose of non-sedating antihistamine up to four times the level recommended in the British National Formulary (BNF). This dosage is unlicensed but may be considered on specialist advice, or by a practitioner with appropriate competence and experience
- Ranitidine may provide additional benefit (*unlicensed indication* – 150 mg twice daily for adults). For more information on ranitidine, see the Members' section of the NMIC website

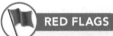

RED FLAGS

- Any suspicion of anaphylaxis (*call 999 immediately; administer adrenaline if available*)
- Suspicion of angioedema (*if significant, treat as anaphylaxis*)
- Unexplained joint pains (*refer to Rheumatology*)
- Children with food allergy trigger (*refer to Allergy Clinic*)
- Pregnant (*see CKS topic Itch in Pregnancy*)
- Painful/persistent (*refer to Dermatology*)
- Antihistamines ineffective (*consider short course [3–5 days] of oral prednisolone[PI], 40 mg/day for adults*)
- Urticaria in children with food allergy triggers may herald future anaphylaxis (*consider referral to Allergy Clinic*)

References

British Association of Dermatologists. 2015. Patient leaflet on urticaria and angioedema. www.bad.org.uk/for-the-public/patient-information-leaflets/urticaria-and-angioedema.

Patient.co.uk. 2016. Urticaria. patient.info/doctor/urticaria-pro.

Powell, R.J., Leech, S.C., Till, S., Huber, P.A.J., Nasser, S.M., and Clark, A.T. 2015. BSACI guideline for the management of chronic urticaria and angioedema. www.bsaci.org/guidelines/chronic-urticaria-and-angioedema.

SCABIES

- Caused by a mite that burrows under the skin, most commonly on the hands (feet in babies). On average, 12 mites are present
- Transmission usually requires prolonged skin contact, although it is thought to be possible through shared towels and bedding. More common in tropical countries (Karimkhani et al., 2014)
- Widespread severe itching, worse at night. May affect the nipples or scrotum
- Sleeping partners or other family members may be affected
- Not acquired from domestic pets (their form of scabies cannot reproduce on humans)
- Common in institutions such as schools, care homes, and nurseries
- Burrows may be visible on hands – bumpy grey lines 2–15 mm long. Skin folds and flexor surfaces are other common sites
- Spreading variable allergic rash usually develops after 2–6 weeks

Self-care

- Permethrin dermal cream should be applied simultaneously to all household and sexual contacts from the previous 2 months. This should be repeated after 7 days. Larger patients may require 2 × 30 g packs. Do not use the liquid 1% creme rinse, which is inadequate for treating scabies
- A prescription is required for babies aged under 2 months (unlicensed indication)
- Despite what the product leaflet may say, apply this to the whole body (BNF 2018), including face, neck, scalp and ears (avoid contact with eyes)
- Be sure to cover finger and toe webs and under nails
- Do not apply just after a bath or shower
- Wash off after 12 hours (i.e. apply in evening and leave on overnight)
- Reapply treatment if washed off before this time (e.g. to hands)
- Machine wash clothes, towels and bedding at high temperature (60°C or above) on day of treatment. Laundry that cannot be washed at a high temperature should be sealed in a plastic bag for at least 72 hours
- Sedating antihistamines (e.g. chlorphenamine[PBI]) give best relief of itch, but sedation may be unacceptable (4 mg at bedtime, repeated after 4 hours if necessary, for adults)
- It is debatable whether non-sedating antihistamines are effective
- Crotamiton[P] may help relieve itch and has some insecticidal activity. Topical corticosteroids may be used once the mites have been eradicated
- If resistant to treatment, then may need referral to Dermatology outpatients for oral ivermectin[PBC]
- **Itching may persist for 6 weeks after mites have been eradicated. It is important that the patient is made aware of this!**

References

BASSH. 2016. UK national guideline on the management of scabies. www.bashhguidelines.org/media/1137/scabies-2016.pdf.

Centers for Disease Control and Prevention. 2010. Scabies frequently asked questions. www.cdc.gov/parasites/scabies/gen_info/faqs.html. *Useful patient information.*

Karimkhani, C., Boyers, L.N., Prescott, L., Welch, V., Delamere, F.M., Nasser, M., Zaveri, A., Hay, R.J., Vos, T., Murray, C.J. and Margolis, D.J. 2014. Global burden of skin disease as reflected in Cochrane Database of Systematic Reviews. *JAMA Dermatol* 150(9):945–951. doi: 10.1001/jamadermatol.2014.709.

PITYRIASIS ROSEA

- Occurs mainly in those aged 10–35, more common in women
- Cause is not known, though herpesvirus 6 and 7 have been implicated (may follow exposure to these)

- Malaise, fever, or lymphadenopathy before the rash appears
- Usually starts with a larger initial 'herald' patch (an oval-shaped area of pink or red scaly skin), often on trunk
- 2–14 days later, the more widespread rash develops with numerous salmon-coloured, oval patches, around 1 cm in diameter, appearing over a period of days. These have a ring of scale on the outer edge
- In people with darker skin, the patches can be grey, brown or black
- Patches line up symmetrically along the dermatomes (see Figure 8.1) on the trunk, face, scalp and upper limbs ('Christmas tree' rash in the T-shirt and shorts area)
- Itching is often present. This is usually mild but may occasionally be intense. Guttate psoriasis affects a similar age group, but the patches are smaller, rounder and pinker

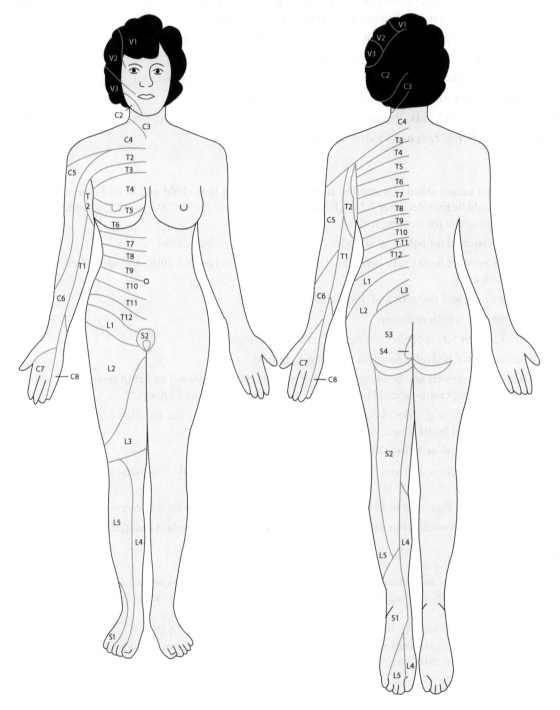

Figure 8.1 Dermatome diagram. Each area is labelled with the spinal nerve that carries sensation from the skin to the spinal cord. The areas overlap to some extent, and an individual person may vary from normal. C: Cervical; L: Lumbar; S: Sacral; T: Thoracic; V: Fifth cranial nerve (trigeminal).

Self-care

- New crops may occur for several weeks
- Rash will last 2–12 weeks then disappear, leaving no trace
- In dark-skinned people, the marks may take longer to fade
- Not contagious
- Unlikely to recur (2%)
- Can try emollients for itching (e.g. hydrous ointment)
- Hydrocortisone ointment if itching severe

RED FLAG

- Pregnant (*concern about miscarriage* [Drago et al., 2014])

References

Chuh, A., Chan, H., and Zawar, V. 2004. Pityriasis rosea–evidence for and against an infectious aetiology. *Epidemiol Infect*; 132(3): 381–390. www.ncbi.nlm.nih.gov/pmc/articles/PMC2870116/. doi: 10.1017/S0950268804002304.

Drago, F., Broccolo, F., Javor, S., Drago, F., Rebora, A., and Parodi A. 2014. Evidence of human herpesvirus-6 and-7 reactivation in miscarrying women with pityriasis rosea. *J Am Acad Dermatol*; 71(1): 198–199. www.jaad.org/article/S0190-9622(14)01140-2/fulltext. doi: 10.1016/j.jaad.2014.02.023.

NICE CKS. 2016. Pityriasis rosea. cks.nice.org.uk/pityriasis-rosea.

RASH IN A SERIOUSLY ILL PATIENT

1. Measles
2. Meningococcal septicaemia

Remember to ask about the travel history in these patients. If recently returned from a tropical area, seek advice from microbiologist or the Hospital for Tropical Diseases (020 3456 7891)

MEASLES

Rare but outbreaks still occur (the number of UK cases varied between 91 and 2030 in the 10 years prior to 2018). Unlikely if two measles, mumps and rubella (MMR) vaccinations have been given.

History

- Incubation period 10 days, infectious for 4 days before, and until 4 days after, onset of rash
- 1–4 days of malaise, loss of appetite, nasal discharge, cough and conjunctivitis
- Rash starts on face and moves down the body
- High fever >39°C starting at onset of rash
- Immunosuppressed
- Pregnant
- Baby under 12 months

Examination

- Koplik's spots may appear just before the rash; blue-grey specks on a red base on the lining of the cheek or gums
- Bright red maculopapular (flat and raised) areas that coalesce and then peel after 5–7 days, starting on face and moving down the body, affecting palms and soles
- Check ears and chest if secondary infection suspected (*may need admission if evidence of pneumonia*)
- Check for signs of dehydration (*consider admission*)

Self-care

- Infectious from 4 days before, to 4 days after, the onset of the rash – stay off work/school and avoid contact with high risk groups (see following section)
- Recovery may take 10 days
- Take paracetamol if needed for muscular pains
- Some national guidelines recommend ibuprofen or paracetamol to relieve symptoms in measles, but in our view there may be a risk in suppressing fever and the immune response to a serious infection
- Drink adequate fluids
- Wash hands frequently. Avoid sharing cutlery, cups and towels; dispose of used tissues immediately

Action

- Notify Health Protection Team
- Exclude from school or work for 4 days after onset of rash
- Saliva tests will probably be requested to confirm the diagnosis. Most people who are suspected of having measles may test negative and have an alternative cause for their symptoms
- Antibiotics are not routinely recommended but may be needed for secondary otitis media or pneumonia
- Consider admission if dehydrated or evidence of pneumonia

RED FLAG

- The following groups are at high risk of complications. If they have had a significant contact with someone with measles, they may need immunoglobulin arranged through the Health Protection Team (see Public Health England, 2017a):
  - Immunosuppressed
  - Pregnant
  - Infant age <1 year

References

Kabra, S.K., and Lodha, R. 2013. Antibiotics for preventing complications in children with measles. *Cochrane Database Syst Rev*; (8): Art. No.: CD001477. doi: 10.1002/14651858.CD001477.pub4.

NICE CKS. 2013. Measles. cks.nice.org.uk/measles.

Public Health England. 2016. Guidance on viral rash in pregnancy. www.gov.uk/government/publications/viral-rash-in-pregnancy.

Public Health England. 2017a. Immunoglobulin: When to use. www.gov.uk/government/publications/immunoglobulin-when-to-use.

Public Health England. 2017b. PHE National Measles Guidelines. www.gov.uk/government/publications/national-measles-guidelines.

MENINGOCOCCAL SEPTICAEMIA

- Rare (the average GP may see two cases in their career) and declining due to vaccination
- 10% mortality
- May occur at any age

Typical Presentation

- The history will be short – hours or days, not weeks
- Patient looks ill, often irritable
- Fever
- Symptoms may be non-specific initially
- They may have flu-like symptoms with sore throat, headache and muscle/joint pain (especially leg pain)
- There may be gastrointestinal symptoms such as nausea, vomiting or diarrhoea
- Any rash: beware that early in the disease this may be macular/papular and only later become petechial
- Confused or drowsy
- Photophobia
- In babies, high-pitched cry

Examination

- The classic sign is neck stiffness, but this is not only found in meningococcal disease. In a relatively well person with discomfort on turning the head, muscular inflammation or tender cervical lymphadenopathy are more likely causes
- Check if the patient can bend the neck fully forwards
- Can a child 'kiss their knees'?
- There are specific techniques to detect meningism (see Box 8.1), but these signs are only apparent when the patient is seriously unwell
- The classic rash is purpuric (dull purplish red macules that do not blanch on pressure), but there may be a non-specific rash in the early stages
- More general signs of sepsis (see Chapter 3) include low blood pressure, rapid pulse, fast respiratory rate, and, in children, a capillary refill time >2 s. Babies may have a stiff body or could be agitated, floppy or unresponsive
- In babies under 3 months with bacterial meningitis, 50% have no fever (Okike et al., 2018)
- Fontanelle (if not yet closed) may be bulging

BOX 8.1 SIGNS OF MENINGISM

Kernig's sign is positive when the thigh is flexed at the hip with the knee at 90 degrees, and subsequent extension in the knee causes pain in the back and neck (leading to resistance).

Brudzinski's sign is positive when lifting a patient's head off the examining couch causes involuntary lifting of the legs.

If suspected:

🚩 Give benzylpenicillin IV/IM (<1 year, 300 mg; 1–9 years, 600 mg; 10 years to adult, 1.2 g) and transfer to hospital by emergency ambulance

References

NICE CG102. 2010. Meningitis (bacterial) and meningococcal septicaemia in under 16s: Recognition, diagnosis and management. www.nice.org.uk/guidance/cg102.

Okike, I.O., Ladhani, S.N., Johnson, A.P., Henderson, K.L., Blackburn, R.M., Muller-Pebody, B., Cafferkey, M., Anthony, M., Ninis, N. and Heath, P.T. 2018. Clinical characteristics and risk factors for poor outcome in infants less than 90 days of age with bacterial meningitis in the United Kingdom and Ireland. *Pediatr Infect Dis J.* journals.lww.com/pidj/Abstract/publishahead/Clinical_Characteristics_and_Risk_Factors_for_Poor.96764.aspx. doi: 10.1097/INF.0000000000001917.

RASH IN A FEBRILE PATIENT

1. Nonspecific viral infection
2. Slapped cheek (parvovirus B19)
3. Hand, foot and mouth disease
4. Scarlet fever

NONSPECIFIC VIRAL INFECTION

Many viruses cause a diffuse macular rash. There are thousands of different types of virus, and the type of rash that they cause is not consistent, so it is usually impossible to name the virus. It may reassure the patient or the parent to know if there have been similar cases in the neighbourhood. Some specific syndromes such as roseola infantum have been described, but in the absence of any specific treatment, such labels are rarely helpful. Usually, it does not matter that you cannot identify the virus, unless the patient is pregnant or has been in contact with a pregnant woman. Rubella is now very rare; there were only two confirmed cases in the United Kingdom in 2016, and pregnant women are no longer being tested for immunity. Parvovirus is much more common.

History

- Often accompanied by symptoms such as runny nose, dry cough, loose stools or fever

Examination

- Check and record temperature, capillary refill (in children), pulse rate and respiratory rate
- Targeted examination based on any symptoms – chest, abdomen, ears
- Consider scarlet fever (see section which follows); if suspected, check throat

Self-care

- No treatment available for nonspecific viral infection, other than supportive measures
- No exclusion from school needed

 RED FLAG

- Pregnant (*see Public Health England, 2016*)

Reference

Public Health England. 2016. Guidance on viral rash in pregnancy. www.gov.uk/government/publications/viral-rash-in-pregnancy.

SLAPPED CHEEK (PARVOVIRUS)

- Also known as erythema infectiosum or Fifth Disease
- Caused by *parvovirus B19*
- Common in children aged 6–10, though may occur at any age; 50% of adults have been infected
- Bright red cheeks
- May have fever, nasal discharge, diarrhoea preceding the onset of the rash
- May be followed by lacy rash on trunk and limbs
- Joint pains in adults
- Immunosuppressed patients may develop bone marrow problems

Self-care

- No specific treatment available
- No exclusion from school needed
- Can take paracetamol or ibuprofen[P] for joint pain

 RED FLAGS

- Pregnant (*may cause miscarriage; inform Obstetrics*)
- Immunosuppressed (*may develop chronic anaemia; check full blood count [FBC] and reticulocytes*)
- Blood disorders (*may develop aplastic anaemia; check FBC and reticulocytes*)

References

NICE CKS. 2017. Parvovirus b19. cks.nice.org.uk/parvovirus-b19.
Public Health England. 2016. Guidance on viral rash in pregnancy. www.gov.uk/government/publications/viral-rash-in-pregnancy.

HAND, FOOT AND MOUTH DISEASE (HFMD)

- Caused by a virus (usually *coxsackie A16*)
- Mainly affects children under 10
- Fever, sore throat, and malaise
- Painful vesicles in mouth, then papules on hands and feet, which turn into vesicles. Groin and buttocks may also be affected
- Not related to foot and mouth disease in animals

Self-care

- No specific treatment available
- No exclusion from school needed
- Take paracetamol or ibuprofen[P] for pain
- Watch fluid intake and seek help if dehydration suspected
- Nails may be shed several months later

RED FLAG

- Pregnant woman with delivery expected within 3 weeks (*low risk of severe illness; discuss with Obstetrics*). Outside this period, reassure the woman that there is no risk to the foetus

References

NICE CKS. 2016. Hand, foot and mouth disease. cks.nice.org.uk/hand-foot-and-mouth-disease.

Ventarola, D., Bordone, L., and Silverberg, N. 2015. Update on hand-foot-and-mouth disease. *Clin Dermatol*; 33(3): 340–346.

SCARLET FEVER

- Caused by group A *Streptococcus* (GABHS)
- Over 17,000 cases in England and Wales in 2016, peaking in February/March
- Commonest in children (peak at age 4)
- Sore throat and cervical lymphadenopathy
- Fever, malaise and headache
- Nausea and vomiting
- Blanching, rough, red pinpricks (which feel like sandpaper) starting on abdomen and chest. Peels after 7 days
- Skin folds deep red in colour
- Flushed face, pale around the mouth
- 'Strawberry tongue' – a white coating may form on the tongue that then peels, leaving a red and swollen tongue
- Red throat with macules over the hard and soft palate
- Complications are rare – invasive streptococcal infection, secondary infections (e.g. pneumonia), late complications (e.g. rheumatic fever, glomerulonephritis). Sepsis is more likely if there is a breach in the skin, e.g. from a wound or co-existing chickenpox

Self-care

- Scarlet fever is generally less serious than it used to be
- Infectious until 24 hours after starting antibiotics – especially avoid contact with immunosuppressed people, those with heart valve problems, open wounds or chickenpox
- Without antibiotics, people remain infectious for up to 3 weeks after symptoms have appeared
- Wash hands frequently; avoid sharing cutlery, cups and towels; put used tissues in bin immediately

Action

- Take a throat swab if the patient is allergic to penicillin, is in contact with vulnerable people, or if an outbreak is suspected
- Prescribe phenoxymethylpenicillin for 10 days (500 mg four times a day for adults). If a child cannot tolerate phenoxymethylpenicillin suspension, use amoxicillin in an unusual dose regime of 50 mg/kg once daily (max 1000 mg) for 10 days
- If allergic to penicillin, use azithromycin[PQ] for 5 days (500 mg once daily for adults)
- Notify Health Protection Team

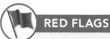

RED FLAGS

- Structural heart disease (*consider admission*)
- Immunosuppressed (*consider admission*)
- At high risk of invasive complications due to, for example, chickenpox, wounds, recent pregnancy (*monitor carefully for sepsis*)

References

NICE CKS. 2015. Scarlet fever. cks.nice.org.uk/scarlet-fever.

Public Health England. 2018. Guidelines for the public health management of scarlet fever outbreaks in schools, nurseries and other childcare settings. PHE Gateway number 2017524. www.gov.uk/government/publications/scarlet-fever-managing-outbreaks-in-schools-and-nurseries

Shulman, S., Bisno, A., Clegg, H., Gerber, M., Kaplan, E., Lee, G., Martin, J., and Van Beneden, C. 2012. Clinical practice guideline for the diagnosis and management of group A streptococcal pharyngitis: 2012 update by the Infectious Diseases Society of America. *Clin Infect Dis*; 55(10): 1279–1282. doi: 10.1093/cid/cis847. *This is the reference given by CKS for a 5-day course of azithromycin and the unusual (in the UK) amoxicillin regime, which are both licensed in the United States for streptococcal throat infections in children.*

PURPLE RASHES

Purple rashes are usually caused by leaking of blood from the vessels just under the skin; therefore, they do not blanch with pressure or when covered by a glass (the 'tumbler test'). Pinpoint rashes are described as petechial, larger areas as purpuric. Such rashes may be caused by:

- Pressure changes, for example, attempted strangulation, violent vomiting, 'love bites'
- Meningococcal septicaemia
- Platelet or clotting abnormalities, for example, leukaemia, thrombocytopenia, aspirin in the elderly
- Vasculitis, for example, Henoch-Schönlein purpura (HSP), which mainly affects children

RED FLAG

- A patient with unexplained purple rash requires urgent assessment (*999 if sepsis suspected, Paediatric assessment for HSP; otherwise an urgent FBC*)

LOCALISED RASHES

1. Cold sores
2. Shingles
3. Warts and verrucae
4. Molluscum contagiosum
5. Fungal infections
6. Nappy rash

COLD SORES

Caused by recurrence of herpes simplex virus (usually HSV-1).

History

- Often recurrent on same site (not always the lip)
- Tingling in skin before appearance of the sore
- Triggers include stress, ultraviolet (UV) light, premenstruation, minor trauma to the area, and other infections such as colds or pneumonia

Examination

- Crops of vesicles on the border of the lip, tongue or mouth that break down into small red areas with yellowish membrane
- Check for evidence of cellulitis (see section on Localised Bacterial Infections)

Self-care

- Aciclovir[P] cream, as soon as possible and certainly within 48 hours of appearance *(not in pregnancy; poor evidence base, and for this indication, the benefit does not outweigh the small risk)*. At first sign of attack, apply to lesions five times a day (approximately every 4 hours), for 5–10 days
- Do not share objects that have touched the area
- Take care not to touch eyes or genitalia after touching cold sore
- Sunblock may help prevention
- Avoid non-essential contact with babies under 4 weeks old until sore has healed (risk of herpes simplex encephalitis). Mothers need to minimise the risk of transferring virus from the cold sore to the baby

Action/prescription

- If immunosuppressed, recurrent or severe symptoms, consider oral aciclovir (400 mg twice daily for adults and children over 12 years) from the time of onset of prodromal symptoms before vesicles appear, if possible, until lesions have healed, for a minimum of 5 days

RED FLAGS

- Immunosuppressed (*at increased risk of complications; discuss with senior colleague*)
- Pregnant and near term (*theoretical risk to baby; discuss with Obstetrics*)

References

Chi, C.C., Wang, S.H., Delamere, F.M., Woinarowska, F., Peters, M.C., and Kanjirath, P.P. 2015. Interventions for prevention of herpes simplex labialis. *Cochrane Database Syst Rev*; (8): CD010095. doi: 10.1002/14651858.CD010095.pub2.
NICE CKS. 2016. Herpes simplex – oral. cks.nice.org.uk/herpes-simplex-oral.

SHINGLES

Caused by recurrence of varicella zoster virus (also called herpes zoster), often after a period of debility or psychosocial stress. Commoner and more likely to cause long-term pain in those over 50. Unlikely to recur – people who have been diagnosed with recurrent shingles in the same area usually have herpes simplex.

History

- Affects area of skin supplied by one nerve root (see Figure 8.1)
- Therefore, only one side of the body is affected. If the rash crosses the midline by more than two thumb-widths, it is not shingles
- Malaise, mild fever, and burning or tingling pain may occur up to 4 days before the rash appears
- Recurrence is rare – if in same area, more likely to be herpes simplex (see previous section)

Examination

- Affects the area of skin supplied by one nerve root (dermatome); commonest on the chest
- Starts with macules and papules that develop into painful vesicles weeping infectious fluid
- They crust over and heal after 2–4 weeks
- Note which nerve root is affected (see Figure 8.1)
- If face is affected, check whether rash involves the eye or the nose
- Local lymph nodes may be enlarged

Self-care

- Keep the rash dry
- Creams and lotions are best avoided because of the risk of spreading skin bacteria into the blistered area
- Adhesive dressings are not recommended
- Infectious until all vesicles have crusted over (usually 5–7 days). Avoid non-essential contact with babies less than 1 month old, pregnant women who have not had chickenpox before, and anyone who is immunosuppressed
- Fluid from the rash cannot give anyone shingles but could give chickenpox to someone who has not had chickenpox before. However, the risk of infection is very low if the rash is covered, and routine exclusion from school and work is not necessary
- Malaise may require rest and time off work
- Seek advice again if the rash flares up or fever develops (this may be secondary bacterial infection needing antibiotics)
- Avoid ibuprofen (increased risk of secondary bacterial infection)

Prescription

- Aciclovir tablets (800 mg five times daily for adults)
- For 7 days if within 72 hours of onset of rash and any of the following:
  - Aged over 50
  - Affecting area other than the trunk
  - Severe symptoms
- For 10 days if:
  - Immunosuppressed (see Red Flags box below)
  - Nose or eye affected – also prescribe aciclovir eye ointment five times daily (and see Red Flags box below)

RED FLAGS

- Nose or eye affected (*prescribe oral and topical aciclovir; refer same-day to Ophthalmology*)
- Immunosuppressed patient with severe symptoms (*may need IV antivirals; seek specialist advice*)
- Pregnant or breastfeeding and eligible for aciclovir (*shingles will not affect the foetus but the risk of antivirals is uncertain; seek specialist advice*)

References

Apok, V., Gurusinghe, N.T., Mitchell, J.D., and Emsley, H.C.A. 2011. Dermatomes and dogma. *Pract Neurol*; 11(2): 100. pn.bmj.com/content/11/2/100.abstract. doi: 10.1136/jnnp.2011.242222.

NICE CKS. 2016. Shingles. cks.nice.org.uk/shingles.

Opstelten, W., and Zaal, M.J.W. 2005. Managing ophthalmic herpes zoster in primary care. *BMJ*; 331(7509): 147–151. www.ncbi.nlm.nih.gov/pmc/articles/PMC558704/. doi: 10.1136/bmj.331.7509.147. *The evidence of benefit of adding in aciclovir eye ointment is insubstantial, but it will produce much higher concentrations of the drug in the anterior eye and provide some lubrication.*

WARTS AND VERRUCAE

- Typical warts are raised pale swellings and may have a surface like a cauliflower
- Verrucae are flattened areas with underlying black dots
- Caused by strains of human papillomavirus (HPV)

Self-care

- Contagious – take steps to avoid self- or cross-infection. People with a verruca should use a waterproof plaster for swimming and avoid sharing towels
- Most disappear by themselves with time but may take 2–3 years
- Avoid scratching or picking them
- Generally best left untreated. See the brief decision aid on Patient.info

- Salicylic acid (OTC) – limited evidence:
  - May cause chemical burns
  - Do not apply to the face
  - Do not use in people with diabetes, peripheral vascular disease or reduced sensation
  - Proper application is important:
    - Remove hard skin with an emery board
    - Soak in warm water for 5–10 minutes
    - Avoid paring or applying the treatment to the surrounding skin
    - Treat daily for at least 12 weeks
- Liquid nitrogen[c] (cryotherapy) – poor evidence:
  - Not for children under the age of 10
  - Not suitable for people with diabetes, poor circulation or reduced sensation
  - May also cause dramatic blood blistering, temporary numbness and scarring
  - 4–6 treatments may be needed
  - OTC products do not lower the skin temperature to the same degree
- Duct tape – limited evidence (de Haen et al., 2006):
  - Cover the wart with duct tape for 6 days
  - If tape falls off, apply a fresh piece
  - Remove tape, soak wart in water, and debride with emery board
  - Leave the wart uncovered overnight and apply a fresh piece of tape next day
  - Continue treatment for up to 2 months
- Banana skin – no evidence:
  - Anecdotally, the application of a banana skin (with the white inside part taped against the wart) each night for 2 weeks has often been reported to be effective, but it seems highly unlikely that a clinical trial on this treatment would ever be funded. It does have the advantage of being virtually free, with no known side effects

RED FLAGS

- Anogenital warts (*refer to Sexual Health*)
- Single wart in the elderly or immunosuppressed (*raised crusted lesion on head/neck/hand may be a squamous carcinoma; 2-week wait skin cancer referral*)

References

de Haen, M., Spigt, M.G., van Uden, C.J., van Neer, P., Feron, F.J., and Knottnerus, A. 2006. Efficacy of duct tape vs placebo in the treatment of verruca vulgaris (warts) in primary school children. *Archives of Pediatrics & Adolescent Medicine*, 160(11), pp. 1121–1125.

Patient.info. 2015. Warts and verrucas – brief decision aid. patient.info/decision-aids/warts-and-verrucas-decision.

Sterling, J.C., Gibbs, S., Haque Hussain, S.S., Mohd Mustapa, M.F., and Handfield-Jones, S.E. 2014. British Association of Dermatologists' guidelines for the management of cutaneous warts. *Br J Dermatol*; 171(4): 696–712. www.bad.org.uk/library-media%5Cdocuments%5CWarts_2014.pdf.

MOLLUSCUM CONTAGIOSUM

This is a poxvirus infection that produces clusters of round, raised, pearly white lesions (sometimes with a darker central dimple) usually on the trunk and limbs of children. It is best left untreated as it resolves completely, without scarring, after several months. If itching is a problem, treat with emollients or hydrocortisone ointment. Sometimes secondary bacterial infection may occur.

Reference

van der Wouden, J.C., van der Sande, R., Kruithof, E.J., Sollie, A., van Suijlekom-Smit, L.W.A., and Koning, S. 2017. Interventions for cutaneous molluscum contagiosum. *Cochrane Database Syst Rev*; (5): Art. No.: CD004767. doi: 10.1002/14651858.CD004767.pub4. *This review found no significant evidence for any intervention, including potassium hydroxide.*

FUNGAL INFECTIONS (TINEA)

Can affect:
- Foot (athlete's foot, tinea pedis)
- Groin (tinea cruris)
- Body (ringworm, tinea corporis)
- Nails (onychomycosis or tinea unguium)

History
- Itchy red rash, slowly spreading over several weeks
- Treatments tried
- Any domestic pets with itchy skin conditions

Examination
- Eczema-like patches
- Not usually symmetrical across the midline
- Often a scaly, inflamed edge
- Central area may appear normal
- May be anywhere on the body; commonly in toe webs, under breasts (intertrigo), in groin
- Affected nails may be thickened and discoloured – usually starting at the edges and spreading inward

Self-care
- Explain that it is an infection acquired from other humans or animals
- Wash the affected area daily and dry thoroughly
- Wash clothes, towels and bed linen frequently
- Wear loose-fitting clothes made of cotton or a material designed to wick moisture away from the skin. For nail infections, wear clean socks every day
- Itchy pets should be checked by a vet
- Terbinafine cream[PBC] (OTC) twice daily for 7–14 days is first line, except in tinea cruris, children *(unlicensed)*, pregnancy or breastfeeding *(poor evidence base, and for this indication, the benefit does not outweigh the small risk)*
- Second line: Clotrimazole cream 1% (OTC) twice daily for 4–6 weeks (continue for 1–2 weeks after rash has resolved)
- Third line: Undecanoic acid cream (OTC) twice daily for 4–6 weeks
- Hydrocortisone 1% cream (OTC) once daily may be added initially to reduce itching
- For nail infections, amorolfine[PBC] 5% nail lacquer (OTC) once weekly for 4–12 months (cure rate only 15%–30%). If successful, the infected nail may not change, but new nail growth (from the base) will appear normal
- Urea and hydrogen peroxide enhance the effect of antifungal medicines on nail infections (Pan et al., 2013). This combination is available in the UK only as an ear drop: Exterol® or Otex® (OTC) *(unlicensed indication)*
- There is some evidence to support using daily application to the nail of Vicks VapoRub® (Derby et al., 2011)

Action
- If rash/nail infection persists despite an adequate course of topical treatment, reconsider diagnosis and take skin scrapings from the scaly edge or nail clippings; oral treatment (e.g. terbinafine) may be needed

Prescription
- Note that NHS England (2018) identified lymphoedema and previous cellulitis as exceptions to the OTC prescribing restrictions

References

British Association of Dermatologists. 2017. Patient leaflet on fungal infections of the nails. www.bad.org.uk/for-the-public/patient-information-leaflets/fungal-infections-of-the-nails.

Derby, R., Rohal, P., Jackson, C., Beutler, A., and Olsen, C. 2011. Novel treatment of onychomycosis using over-the-counter mentholated ointment: A clinical case series. *Am Board Fam Med*; 24(1): 69–77. *The ingredients in Vicks VapoRub (thymol, menthol, camphor, and oil of eucalyptus) have shown efficacy against dermatophytes in vitro. 83% of the 18 participants in this trial had a positive response.*

Kreijkamp-Kaspers, S., Hawke, K., Guo, L., Kerin, G., Bell-Syer, SEM., Magin, P., Bell-Syer, S.V. et al. 2017. Oral antifungal medication for toenail onychomycosis. Cochrane Database of Systematic Reviews Issue 7. Art. No.: CD010031. doi: 10.1002/14651858.CD010031. pub2. *Terbinafine had the best cure rate and side effect profile*

NHS England. 2018. Conditions for which over the counter items should not routinely be prescribed in primary care: Guidance for CCGs. www.england.nhs.uk/publication/conditions-for-which-over-the-counter-items-should-not-routinely-be-prescribed-in-primary-care-guidance-for-ccgs/

Pan, M., Heinecke, G., Bernardo, S., Tsui, C., and Levitt, J. 2013. Urea: A comprehensive review of the clinical literature. *Dermatol Online J;* 19(11). http://escholarship.org/uc/item/11×463rp. *Combination therapies consisting of urea with a variety of antifungal agents have been found to partially cure onychomycosis in some patients. By softening the nail bed, urea facilitates greater penetration of antifungal medicines.*

Public Health England. 2017. Fungal skin and nail infections: Diagnosis and laboratory investigation. www.gov.uk/government/uploads/system/uploads/attachment_data/file/619770/Fungal_skin_and_nail_infections_guidance.pdf.

NAPPY RASH

History

- Duration
- Type of nappy, changing routine, cleansers used
- Distress on changing nappy
- Creams already tried
- Other areas affected (makes nappy rash unlikely)

Examination

- Red and shiny or scaly areas
- Check for satellite spots
- Look for oral thrush, which often co-exists (and treat if found)

Self-care

- Leave nappy off when possible
- Clean and change nappy as soon as wet or soiled
- Use water or fragrance-free and alcohol-free baby wipes
- Dry gently after cleaning – avoid vigorous rubbing
- Bathe once daily
- Do not use soap or bath additives. Consider soap substitute, for example, Hydromol Bath and Shower® (OTC)
- Use high-absorbency nappies
- Barrier creams should not be used routinely as they can prevent the nappy from absorbing liquid away from the skin, but if rash is present, apply one such as Metanium® (OTC) or dexpanthenol 5% (OTC) at each nappy change
- Fungal infection is common in nappy rash that has been present for more than 48 hours. The presence of satellite spots, distress, and the involvement of the skin creases make this more likely. If suspected, recommend clotrimazole 1% cream for 3 weeks and avoid barrier cream

RED FLAG

- Secondary bacterial infection is rare (*if suspected, take swab and prescribe flucloxacillin or, if allergic to penicillin, clarithromycin[PIQ]*)
- Primary streptococcal proctitis may cause severe inflammation around the anus (*if suspected, take swab and prescribe amoxicillin or, if allergic to penicillin, clarithromycin[PIQ]*)

References

Bonifaz, A., Rojas, R., Tirado-Sánchez, A., Chávez-López, D., Mena, C., Calderón, L., and María, P.R. 2016. Superficial mycoses associated with diaper dermatitis. *Mycopathologia;* 181: 671–679. link.springer.com/article/10.1007%2Fs11046-016-0020-9. doi: 10.1007/s11046-016-0020-9.

Cohen, R., Levy, C., Bonacorsi, S., Wollner, A., Koskas, M., Jung, C., Béchet, S., Chalumeau, M., Cohen, J., and Bidet, P. 2015. Diagnostic accuracy of clinical symptoms and rapid diagnostic test in group A streptococcal perianal infections in children. *Clin Infect Dis;* 60(2): 267–270. academic.oup.com/cid/article-lookup/doi/10.1093/cid/ciu794. doi: 10.1093/cid/ciu794.

LOCALISED BACTERIAL INFECTIONS

1. Impetigo
2. Boils
3. Cellulitis
4. Ingrowing toenail
5. Paronychia

IMPETIGO

- Golden crusted lesions of the superficial skin, usually caused by *Staphylococcus*, sometimes *Streptococcus*
- Typically 2 cm in diameter, resembling 'glued-on cornflakes'
- Commonly on faces of children, though may occur elsewhere
- May be secondary to wound or viral lesion
- Patient may be systemically unwell if infection is severe
- Bullous impetigo (blistering and painful) is uncommon; neonates are most often affected

Self-care

- Will heal without scarring, unless picked
- Wash off crusts with soapy water
- Stay out of school until lesions crusted or for 48 hours after starting treatment
- Do not share face cloths or towels
- Topical antiseptics have been suggested as an alternative to topical antibiotics because of concerns about antibiotic resistance, but evidence is lacking

Prescription

- Topical sodium fusidate ointment for 7–10 days, if localised
- Consider treating inside nostrils with Naseptin® if recurrent facial impetigo
- Send swab for culture if not responding to treatment
- Retapamulin ointment, twice daily for 5 days, is second line if resistance to fusidic acid is suspected
- Prescribe oral flucloxacillin for 7 days (250–500 mg four times daily for adults) if bullous, extensive, severe, or spreading despite topical treatment (or clarithromycin[PIQ] 250–500 mg twice daily for adults if the patient is allergic to penicillin)
- Do not use mupirocin, which should be reserved for treatment of methicillin-resistant *Staphylococcus aureus* (MRSA)
- Advise patient to seek help if worsening or no improvement after 7 days

References

Chaplin, S. 2016. Topical antibacterial and antiviral agents: Prescribing and resistance. *Prescriber*; 27: 29–36. onlinelibrary.wiley.com/doi/10.1002/psb.1480/pdf.
NICE CKS. 2015. Impetigo. cks.nice.org.uk/impetigo.
Thomas, M. 2017. Topical antibiotics for skin infections: When are they appropriate? Best Practice Advocacy Centre New Zealand. www.bpac.org.nz/2017/topical-antibiotics-2.aspx.

BOILS AND CARBUNCLES

A boil is an infection of a single hair follicle, usually caused by *Staphylococcus aureus*. A carbuncle is a larger lesion caused by several boils joining together. It is more painful than a boil, and the patient may be systemically unwell.

History

- Duration
- Fever or pain
- Discharge

- Are these recurrent?
- Any contacts with similar boils?
- Risk factors (see later) and/or symptoms of diabetes: thirst/polyuria/tiredness
- Immunosuppressed

Examination

- Fluctuation (sensation of fluid moving between two fingers placed on either side – imagine a balloon full of water)
- Cellulitis – is the surrounding skin hot, red and tender?
- Enlarged lymph nodes (suggest underlying cellulitis)

Tests

If the infection is recurrent, severe or affecting other family members:

- Swab lesion, nose and axilla, to identify staphylococcal carriage (affects around 20% of population, commoner in healthcare workers), and ask the lab to check for Panton-Valentine leucocidin *Staphylococcus aureus* (PVL-SA) (for more information see BAD 2016 reference)
- Check for immunosuppression:
  - Full blood count
  - Fasting plasma glucose or HbA1c (see Box 8.2)
  - Consider HIV test

BOX 8.2 CHECKING FOR DIABETES

Much has been written about this, and there will be a protocol for your area based on the international criteria for diagnosis and the characteristics of the various tests for diabetes. The protocol might start with a fasting plasma glucose level or HbA1c as the first step, but screening whole populations in this way is burdensome and not as effective as targeting those at higher risk of diabetes. But how do you decide who is at high risk?

- Suspected diabetes: If you strongly suspect diabetes because of classic symptoms, such as thirst, polyuria and weight loss, then urgent testing with fasting plasma glucose (and HbA1c) is needed. Only one diabetes-range result is needed in this situation to make the diagnosis (i.e. you do not need to repeat testing). Remember, HbA1c is not reliable in pregnancy or any condition affecting blood cell turnover (such as anaemia), and may be normal in new-onset Type 1 diabetes. Follow your local protocol. Testing capillary blood glucose during the consultation can also be useful (although venous testing is still necessary to make the diagnosis) – a result of over 15 mmol/l should prompt referral to a senior colleague.
- High risk: If the patient is at high risk of having diabetes but has no classic symptoms, follow your local protocol for testing (either fasting plasma glucose or HbA1c if clinically appropriate). Without the osmotic symptoms of thirst or polyuria, any diabetes-range results should be repeated to confirm the diagnosis. The main risk factors include positive family history, South Asian or African-Caribbean ethnicity, being a male over 40, being overweight or obese, being physically inactive, having a background of high blood pressure, previous gestational diabetes or current anti-psychotic medication. The Diabetes UK Know Your Risk tool, found at https://riskscore.diabetes.org.uk/, is useful for ascertaining risk – a score of 16 or above suggests high risk.
- Low risk: If the patient has a minor illness known to be more common in those with diabetes, such as cystitis or boils, but has no symptoms of diabetes or significant risk factors, then test the urine for glucose. If this proves positive, then it is quite likely that the patient does indeed have diabetes, but this needs verification with blood tests (and further repeat blood tests for confirmation). If the urine is negative for glucose, this does not completely exclude diabetes (the elderly may not show glucose in the urine despite high blood levels), but the test is adequate when the chance of diabetes is low.

Testing the urine for glucose is useful in primary care when the individual's risk of diabetes is low. The test is quick, inexpensive, does not require the patient to fast, and the result is known immediately. Positive results need further investigation to establish the diagnosis.

Reference

NICE PH38. 2017. Type 2 diabetes: Prevention in people at high risk. www.nice.org.uk/guidance/38.

Self-care

- Apply heat to encourage pointing (e.g. warm flannel) four times daily
- Cover with sterile gauze
- Wash hands after touching the boil
- Do not share towels or flannels
- Wash and tumble dry bedding, towels and underclothes daily
- Avoid swimming until healed
- If getting frequent boils, consider decolonisation treatment with chlorhexidine 4% body wash daily for 5 days (and use as shampoo on days 1, 3, and 5)

Action

- Magnesium sulphate paste is traditionally used, although there is a lack of evidence to support it
- Incise and drain if fluctuant (*refer to Surgical if necessary*)
- Advise patient to watch for symptoms of cellulitis
- Prescribe antibiotic if indicated (see Box 8.3)
- Treat nasal colonisation topically according to swab (mupirocin reserved for MRSA)

 BOX 8.3   ANTIBIOTIC FOR BOILS

Prescribe an antibiotic if:

- Unwell with fever or cellulitis
- High-risk group (immunosuppressed, diabetes)
- On the face
- Carbuncle

Antibiotic choice

If a swab was taken, treat according to sensitivity. If MRSA or PVL-SA isolated, these need special treatment. Take advice from microbiologist. Otherwise:

- Flucloxacillin for 7 days (500 mg four times daily for adults)
- Clarithromycin[PIQ] if the patient is allergic to penicillin (500 mg twice daily for adults)

 RED FLAGS

- Facial boil causing cellulitis (*can be life-threatening; admit under Medical or Paediatrics*)
- Apparent boil in anogenital area or natal cleft (between buttocks) (*may be Bartholin's cyst, Crohn's disease or pilonidal abscess; consider referral to Surgical or Gynaecology*)
- Fluctuant boil requiring incision and drainage in surgical high-risk area: face, neck, axilla, groin (*refer same-day to Surgical*)

References

British Association of Dermatologists. 2016. Panton-Valentine leucocidin Staphylococcus aureus information leaflet. www.bad.org.uk/shared/get-file.ashx?id=179&itemtype=document.

NICE CKS. 2017. Boils, carbuncles, and staphylococcal carriage. cks.nice.org.uk/boils-carbuncles-and-staphylococcal-carriage.

CELLULITIS

A bacterial infection of the deeper layers of the skin, usually caused by *Streptococcus pyogenes* (two-thirds of cases) or *Staphylococcus aureus* (one-third of cases). A potentially serious infection that may lead to sepsis.

History

- Duration
- Nature of any wound or break in the skin
- Pain
- Unilateral localised swelling and heat
- ⚑ Fever/malaise/rigors
- ⚑ Immunosuppression (especially intravenous substance use or diabetes)

Examination

- Temperature, pulse rate and blood pressure
- Well-defined area is red, hot, swollen, hard and tender, with possible vesicles
- Discharge
- Lymphadenopathy
- ⚑ Tracking (lymphangitis)

Tests

- Take swab of any discharge
- If history of recurrent skin infections, or symptoms/risk factors of diabetes, consider blood testing (fasting plasma glucose or HbA1c where suitable)

Self-care

- Keep limb elevated (if applicable)
- Mark boundary with indelible, disposable pen – ask the patient to seek help if area is enlarging beyond boundary
- Take paracetamol for pain
- Use an emollient after 48 hours

Action

- Admit to hospital if any red flags (see list that follows)
- Assess the severity using the Eron score (see Table 8.1)
- Check portal of entry. Wound cleaning and dressing as appropriate
- If patient has diabetes, optimise diabetic control
- Antibiotics for 7–14 days (longer in lymphoedema) (see Table 8.2)

Table 8.1 The Eron classification system for cellulitis

Class I	Systemically well, no uncontrolled co-morbidity
Class II	Systemically unwell or co-morbidity (e.g. peripheral arterial disease, chronic venous insufficiency, or morbid obesity)
Class III	Significant systemic upset, for example, acute confusion, tachycardia, tachypnoea, hypotension, or unstable co-morbidity
Class IV	Sepsis or necrotising fasciitis

Table 8.2 Antibiotic choice for cellulitis

Presentation	Antibiotic	Penicillin allergy
Class I cellulitis	Flucloxacillin (full dose)	Clarithromycin[PIQ]
Class II cellulitis	Consider IV antibiotic (consult microbiologist)	Consider IV antibiotic (consult microbiologist)
Lymphoedema	Amoxicillin. Add flucloxacillin if staph suspected	Clarithromycin[PIQ]
Post chickenpox	Flucloxacillin + amoxicillin	Clarithromycin[PIQ]
Facial cellulitis	Co-amoxiclav	Clarithromycin[PIQ]
Following wound in water	Consult microbiologist	Consult microbiologist

- Review after 48 hours
- If recurrent cellulitis, consider prophylactic antibiotic (Dalal et al., 2017)

Doses for adults

- Flucloxacillin 500 mg four times daily
- Clarithromycin[PIQ] 500 mg twice daily
- Amoxicillin 500 mg three times daily
- Co-amoxiclav 500/125 mg three times daily

RED FLAGS

Consider admission if:

- Class III or IV or rapidly deteriorating cellulitis
- Under 1 year of age or frail
- Immunosuppressed (*especially poorly controlled diabetes*) or at high risk (*e.g. artificial joint*)
- Significant lymphoedema
- Facial cellulitis (*unless very mild*)
- Lymphangitis (*'tracking'*)
- Pointing abscess (*needs incision and drainage/referral to Surgical*)
- Worsening despite treatment or not responding to initial treatment after 3 days

References

Aebi, C., Ahmed, A., and Ramilo, O. 1996. Bacterial complications of primary varicella in children. *Clin Infect Dis*; 23(4): 698–705. http://europepmc.org/abstract/MED/8909829?europe_pmc_extredirect=doi.org/10.1093/clinids/23.4.698. doi: 10.1093/clinids/23.4.698. *The most likely cause of secondary infection of chickenpox is group A beta-hemolytic Streptococcus (59% of cases), with Staphylococcus aureus being the second most likely (28%).*

Dalal, A., Eskin-Schwartz, M., Mimouni, D., Ray, S., Days, W., Hodak, E., Leibovici, L., and Paul, M. 2017. Interventions for the prevention of recurrent erysipelas and cellulitis. *Cochrane Database Syst Rev*; (6): Art. No.: CD009758. doi: 10.1002/14651858.CD009758.pub2. *For people with at least two episodes of cellulitis in the previous 3 years, antibiotic prophylaxis (usually phenoxymethylpenicillin 250 mg twice daily) reduces the number of recurrences by 50%.*

NICE CKS. 2015. Cellulitis – acute. cks.nice.org.uk/cellulitis-acute.

Peterson, D., McLeod, S., Woolfrey, K., and McRae, A. 2014. Predictors of failure of empiric outpatient antibiotic therapy in emergency department patients with uncomplicated cellulitis. *Acad Emerg Med*; 21: 526–531. http://onlinelibrary.wiley.com/doi/10.1111/acem.12371/full. doi: 10.1111/acem.12371. *Fever, leg ulcers, chronic oedema or lymphoedema, prior cellulitis in the same area, and cellulitis at wound site were associated with failure of initial oral antibiotic therapy in American ED patients with cellulitis.*

Phoenix, G., Das, S., and Joshi, M. 2012. Diagnosis and management of cellulitis. *BMJ*; 345. www.bmj.com/content/345/bmj.e4955.abstract. doi: 10.1136/bmj.e4955.

Raff, A.B., and Kroshinsky, D. 2016. Cellulitis: A review. *JAMA*; 316(3): 325–337. http://infectoemicroconsult.com.br/arquivos/Cellulitis.pdf. doi: 10.1001/jama.2016.8825.

INGROWING TOENAIL

History

- Duration
- Discharge
- Previous episodes
- Background/symptoms/risk factors for diabetes

Examination

- Check for evidence of cellulitis – pus, spreading redness or fever
- Inflammation where the nail digs in does not indicate infection
- Discharge
- Granulation tissue

Test

- Swab any discharge

Self-care

- Soak toe in warm salty water for 10 minutes (1 teaspoon of salt in 500 ml water)
- With cotton bud, push skin fold down and away from ingrown nail. Start at root of the nail and move outwards
- Repeat daily for a few weeks
- As end of nail grows forward, push tiny pledget of cotton wool under it to help nail grow over skin
- Change cotton wool daily
- Allow nail to grow forward until clear of end of toe
- Cut nail straight across
- See chiropodist if persistent/recurrent
- Keep feet clean and dry and let air get to toes when possible
- Avoid tight shoes and use cotton socks rather than synthetics

Action

If localised cellulitis (pus, fever, spreading redness):

- Flucloxacillin for 7 days (500 mg four times daily for adults) or, if allergic to penicillin, clarithromycin[PIQ] (500 mg twice daily for adults)

 RED FLAG

- Immunosuppressed or diabetic patient with cellulitis (*consider admission*)

Reference

Harding, M. 2015. Ingrowing toenails. patient.info/health/ingrowing-ingrown-toenails.

PARONYCHIA

- A superficial infection of the skin fold around a nail, usually caused by Staphylococcus
- Pain and swelling at the side/base of one finger
- Nail fold is red, hot, tender and swollen. Pus may be seen
- Check for signs of cellulitis (see previous section)
- If fluctuant, consider incision and drainage
- Advise moist warm compresses three times daily
- Prescribe antibiotic for 7 days: flucloxacillin (250 mg four times daily for adults) or, if allergic to penicillin, clarithromycin[PIQ] (250 mg twice daily for adults) if:
  - Immunosuppressed
  - Fever
  - Non-fluctuant
- Chronic paronychia (develops slowly and lasts for weeks) often needs treatment with antifungal medication

Reference

NICE CKS. 2015. Paronychia – acute. cks.nice.org.uk/paronychia-acute.

MISCELLANEOUS

1. Eczema
2. Seborrhoeic dermatitis
3. Guttate psoriasis
4. Head lice

5. Suspected skin cancer

6. Umbilical granuloma

7. Acne

ECZEMA

This condition accounts for 30% of all skin consultations in primary care. It occurs when the lipid layer that covers the skin becomes thin, causing water loss. A genetically determined deficiency in filaggrin, a protein in the skin, significantly increases the risk of eczema. Emotional or environmental factors may trigger a flare. It is a long-term, relapsing condition; it is important for the patient to appreciate this. The term 'dermatitis' is used for eczema due to a known trigger.

History

- Duration
- Previous episodes
- Suspected cause/trigger (e.g. solvents, nickel, detergents, latex)
- Distribution (usually symmetrical – flexures, face, hands)
- Itching (if absent, eczema is unlikely)
- Previous treatments and effects
- Occupation (hairdressers are at high risk)
- 🚩 Fever/discharge/pain/blisters (suggest infection)

Examination

- Poorly defined inflamed scaly patches
- May be dry and cracking
- Usually symmetrical
- In babies, mainly on the face, or outside surface of elbows and knees. In children and adults, mainly in the flexures (inside surface of elbows and knees)
- Scratch marks/damage/thickening
- 🚩 Portal of entry for infection
- 🚩 Inflamed/weeping/blistered/signs of cellulitis

Tests

- Swab if discharging
- Scrapings for fungal testing if diagnosis in doubt, or treatment unsuccessful

Self-care

- Treatments can control but not cure. In children, usually improves with time
- Avoid scratching – rub with fingertips or soft paintbrush
- Keep cool and avoid synthetic fibres
- Dietary changes and dust mite avoidance are not recommended
- Use emollients (commonly called moisturisers) three or four times daily. Most effective after a bath or shower ('soak and smear'). Stroke them on liberally, do not rub in. Emollients should be obtained OTC for mild irritant dermatitis or mild dry skin
- About 600 g of emollient per week may be needed. It should still be used even when the skin has cleared
- There is no evidence to favour one type of emollient, but patients often have strong preferences. Oilatum® or Cetraben® would be reasonable first choices – be guided by your local formulary. Do not recommend aqueous cream, which may cause skin irritation
- Offer trial sizes first to avoid expensive mistakes
- Tubes or pump dispensers are preferred to pots to avoid contamination from fingers
- Ointments work better than creams, if greasiness tolerated

- Emollients which contain paraffin are flammable. For smokers, or those with high-risk occupations, consider a low paraffin preparation (licensed – see PrescQIPP reference) or a paraffin-free colloidal oat cream, for example, AproDerm Colloidal Oat Cream® (*unlicensed*)
- Do not routinely recommend emollients containing additives (e.g. urea, antiseptic)
- Many emollients may be used as soap substitutes, or these may be bought separately, for example, Hydromol Bath and Shower®
- Bath additives are ineffective (Santer et al., 2018)
- Avoid detergents (e.g. bubble bath – even if marketed for babies). If hands are affected, use cotton-lined rubber gloves for washing-up
- If itching is troublesome, consider chlorphenamine[PBI] at night (4 mg at bedtime, repeated after 4 hours if necessary, for adults)
- Non-sedating antihistamines are unlikely to be effective

Action

- If not responding, reconsider diagnosis (may be fungal) and consider a reaction to sensitiser in emollient. See Box 8.4 for further management
- If infected, prescribe oral flucloxacillin for 7 days (250–500 mg four times daily for adults) or, if allergic to penicillin, clarithromycin[PIQ] (250–500 mg twice daily for adults). Do not use topical antibiotics

---

BOX 8.4   TREATING FLARES OF ECZEMA

- Check for infection
- Use a topical steroid ointment (Eumovate® or hydrocortisone 1%) once daily until 48 hours after the redness has settled
- Fingertip units are a useful measure
- Allow emollient to absorb before applying steroids
- Topical steroids stronger than hydrocortisone may cause atrophy and thinning of the skin after prolonged use. Tiny blood vessels become visible, for which no treatment is available. The skin of the face is the most sensitive, the palms and soles least sensitive. Children's skin is more sensitive than adults' – **do not use any stronger steroid than hydrocortisone 1% in children or on the face** (see Table 8.3)
- Topical steroids can be used in pregnancy and breastfeeding but aim to use the lowest potency steroid to the smallest area of skin necessary and if breastfeeding, either avoid application to the nipple area or clean thoroughly prior to nursing
- 1% hydrocortisone cream should generally be bought OTC (for considerably less than the prescription charge), but the packs carry warnings not to use the product on children under 10, pregnant women, on the face or genital area, and the pharmacist is not allowed to sell them for these purposes. If the patient has been assessed by a clinician and a prescription issued, these warnings no longer apply but the pharmacist is still not permitted to sell the medicine OTC
- Arrange a review appointment to step down treatment

Table 8.3 Topical preparations for eczema

Preparation	Steroid potency
Emollients	Zero
Hydrocortisone 1%	Low
Eumovate®	Moderate
Betnovate®	High

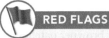 **RED FLAGS**

- Bacterial infection of eczema (*requires prompt antibiotic treatment*)
- Eczema herpeticum is a rare but life-threatening herpes virus infection. It usually affects the head and neck area of a child with eczema and presents with areas of rapidly worsening, painful eczema with clustered vesicles and small, uniform, punched-out erosions. The child may be feverish and distressed (*admit to Paediatrics*)

References

Apfelbacher, C., van Zuuren, E., Fedorowicz, Z., Jupiter, A., Matterne, U., and Weisshaar E. 2013. Oral H1 antihistamines as monotherapy for eczema. *Cochrane Database Syst Rev*; (2): Art. No.: CD007770. doi: 10.1002/14651858.CD007770.pub2. *There is no good evidence of the effectiveness of antihistamines in eczema.*

Baron, S.E., Cohen, S.N., and Archer, C.B. 2012. Guidance on the diagnosis and clinical management of atopic eczema. *Clin Exp Dermatol*; 37(s1): 7–12. http://onlinelibrary.wiley.com/doi/10.1111/j.1365-2230.2012.04336.x/abstract. doi: 10.1111/j.1365-2230.2012.04336.x.

Cardona, I.D., Stillman, L., and Jain, N. 2016. Does bathing frequency matter in pediatric atopic dermatitis? *Ann Allergy Asthma Immunol*; 117(1): 9–13. www.annallergy.org/article/S1081-1206(16)30264-2/abstract. doi: 10.1016/j.anai.2016.05.014. *No strong evidence, but daily bathing is probably best, if used with "soak and smear" emollients.*

Francis, N.A., Ridd, M.J., Thomas-Jones, E., Butler, C.C., Hood, K., Shepherd, V., Marwick, C.A., Huang, C., Longo, M., Wootton, M., Sullivan, F. 2017. Oral and topical antibiotics for clinically infected eczema in children: a pragmatic randomized controlled trial in ambulatory care. *The Annals of Family Medicine*; 15(2): 124–30. *Surprisingly, this trial found no benefit for the use of antibiotics in mildly infected eczema.*

Li, A.W., Yin, E.S., and Antaya, R.J. 2017. Topical corticosteroid phobia in atopic dermatitis, a systematic review. *JAMA Dermatol*; 153(10): 1036–1042. doi: 10.1001/jamadermatol.2017.2437. *Negative feelings and beliefs about topical steroids are common and lead to undertreatment.*

MHRA. 2013. Aqueous cream: May cause skin irritation, particularly in children with eczema, possibly due to sodium lauryl sulfate content. *Drug Safety Update*; 6(8): A2. www.mhra.gov.uk/Safetyinformation/DrugSafetyUpdate/CON254804.

NHS Central Alert System (CAS) reference Rapid Response Report 4. 2007. www.nrls.npsa.nhs.uk/resources/?EntryId45=59876. *Useful patient leaflet and video about fire hazard with emollients.*

Santer, M., Ridd, M.J., Francis, N.A., Stuart, B., Rumsby, K., Chorozoglou, M., Becque, T., Roberts, A., Liddiard, L., Nollett, C., and Hooper, J. 2018. Emollient bath additives for the treatment of childhood eczema (BATHE): multicentre pragmatic parallel group randomised controlled trial of clinical and cost effectiveness. *BMJ* 361, p.k1332. doi.org/10.1136/bmj.k1332.

Smith, K. 2013. Cost effective emollients with no, or low paraffin content. NHS PrescQIPP. *Bulletin* 49: v2.0. www.prescqipp.info/resources/send/92-cost-effective-emollients-with-no-or-low-paraffin-content/1306-bulletin-49-cost-effective-emollients-with-no-or-low-paraffin-content.

van Zuuren, E.J., Fedorowicz, Z., Christensen, R., Lavrijsen, A.P.M., and Arents, B.W.M. 2017. Emollients and moisturisers for eczema. *Cochrane Database Syst Rev*; (2): Art. No.: CD012119. doi: 10.1002/14651858.CD012119.pub2. *No clear evidence to favour any type of emollient.*

SEBORRHOEIC DERMATITIS

This is a type of skin inflammation in areas with many sebaceous glands. It occurs in babies aged 2 weeks to 6 months and in children and adults. It is affected by hormone balance and stress, but the yeast *Malassezia* is also implicated.

- In adults: scalp (dandruff is the non-inflamed form), nasolabial folds, ears, eyebrows and chest
- In infants: scalp (cradle cap), face, ears, neck and nappy area
- Red, flaky, greasy patches that may be itchy

Self-care

- Use emollient soap substitutes, for example, Hydromol Bath and Shower®
- On the skin, use an azole cream, for example, clotrimazole 1% OTC – two to three times daily for at least 4 weeks
- On the scalp, for infants, apply warm olive oil or baby oil and keep on for several hours, then wash with a coal–tar shampoo and brush gently to remove scales. In adults and children over 12 years, ketoconazole[c] 2% shampoo may be used (for at least 4 weeks)

Action

- If self-care measures have failed, review diagnosis and consider adding hydrocortisone 1% ointment

Reference

Harding, M. 2016. Seborrhoeic dermatitis. patient.info/doctor/seborrhoeic-dermatitis-pro.

GUTTATE PSORIASIS

Psoriasis is a common long-term inflammatory condition affecting the skin, joints and nails. Most forms do not present acutely, but guttate psoriasis may mimic other acute rashes, for example, pityriasis rosea (which has larger, browner patches). Guttate psoriasis usually starts in children or young adults and may develop 2–3 weeks after a streptococcal or viral infection.

- Small (<1 cm) round or oval, scaly papules that may be pink or red
- Many scattered lesions, mainly on the trunk and upper limbs
- May also occur on the face, ears and scalp

- Usually resolves spontaneously but may take 3–4 months
- Emollients and topical steroids may improve itching
- Antibiotic treatment is of no benefit

Reference

NICE CKS. 2014. Guttate psoriasis. cks.nice.org.uk/psoriasis#!scenario:3.

HEAD LICE

Common in children, this infestation requires head-to-head contact for transmission.

History

- Nits (hatched egg cases)
- Lice seen
- Scratching
- Outbreaks at schools/institutions

Examination

- Examine head for nits and live lice using a detection plastic comb, for example, Bug Buster®
- Louse eggs adhere to hair tightly, whereas dandruff falls off easily
- Look for enlarged occipital lymph nodes

Self-care

- Check all of household and treat only those in whom live lice have been found
- Wet combing with conditioner is the best method of checking because it immobilises the lice
- Use one of the following methods (all should be obtained OTC):
    - First-line: Dimeticone lotion – best evidence of effectiveness, and resistance is unlikely because of its mode of action (apply once weekly for two doses, rub into dry hair and scalp, allow to dry naturally, shampoo after minimum 8 hours or overnight)
    - Wet combing using the Bug Buster® comb
    - Malathion[B] 0.5% aqueous liquid (apply once weekly for two doses, rub into dry hair and scalp, allow to dry naturally, shampoo after minimum 12 hours)
- Repeat according to method
- Reassure – lice prefer clean hair
- Warn patient that eggs may still be visible after treatment

Reference

NICE CKS. 2016. Head lice. cks.nice.org.uk/head-lice.

SUSPECTED SKIN CANCER

Most moles develop in early childhood and adolescence, and there is a gradual decrease in their number in old age. Not unreasonably, malignant melanoma is a concern behind many consultations, for which most patients need reassurance. Many lesions which patients call moles are, in fact, seborrhoeic keratoses that are superficial (appearing stuck-on), golden brown in colour with a scaly, greasy surface. They are harmless and, in contrast to true moles, are much more common in the elderly.

Not all skin cancers are pigmented. Basal cell carcinomas (rodent ulcers) are pearly lesions most commonly found on the face, whereas squamous cell carcinomas are usually raised and crusted and are typically found on the head, neck or hand of an immunosuppressed patient.

History

- Patient's concerns
- Duration
- Itch/change in sensation
- Inflammation/oozing

- Family history
- History of significant sun exposure
- 🚩 Enlarging/changing shape/changing colour/new mole (70% of melanomas arise in a new mole)
- 🚩 Scabbing over but not healing
- 🚩 Immunosuppressed (*increased risk of squamous cell carcinoma*)
- 🚩 Pigmented lesion under a nail without history of trauma (see Box 8.5)

BOX 8.5 MELANOMA UNDER THE NAIL MAY PRESENT WITH:

- Spreading brown or black streaks in the nail without any known injury
- Bruise on the nail that does not heal or move up as the nail grows
- Nails that thin, crack, distort or separate from the nail bed
- Darkening skin next to the nail
- A nail that bleeds or develops a nodule

Examination

- Colour
- Diameter
- 🚩 Feel for induration (hardness)
- 🚩 Ulceration
- 🚩 Rolled edge may suggest basal cell carcinoma
- 🚩 Small visible blood vessels on surface (easily seen with illuminated magnification) – associated with basal cell carcinoma
- 🚩 Scaling/crusting with red base – suspicious of squamous cell carcinoma
- 🚩 Major features of mole (two points each – see Red Flags box for interpretation):
  - Change in size
  - Irregular shape
  - Irregular colour
- 🚩 Minor features of mole (one point each – see Red Flags box for interpretation):
  - Largest diameter 7 mm or more
  - Inflammation
  - Oozing
  - Change in sensation

Self-care

- Advise the patient to watch the area, ideally measure or photograph it, and seek help if they notice any of the following (ABCDE):
  - Asymmetrical
  - Border irregular
  - Colours (more than one)
  - Diameter (more than 6 mm)
  - Elevated

 RED FLAGS

- Pigmented lesion scoring ≥ 3 points (*2-week wait cancer referral*)
- New lesion in immunosuppressed patient (*2-week wait cancer referral*)
- Suspected squamous cell carcinoma (*2-week wait cancer referral*)
- Suspected basal cell carcinoma (*routine referral to Dermatology*)
- Pigmented lesion under a nail (*2-week wait cancer referral*)

References

Nall, R. 2017. Subungual melanoma: Symptoms, risk factors and treatment. www.medicalnewstoday.com/articles/319100.php.

NICE NG12. 2015. Suspected cancer: Recognition and referral. www.nice.org.uk/guidance/ng12/chapter/1-Recommendations-organised-by-site-of-cancer#skin-cancers.

Pampena, R., Kyrgidis, A., Lallas, A., Moscarella, E., and Argenziano, G. 2017. A meta-analysis of nevus-associated melanoma: Prevalence and practical implications. *JAAD*. www.jaad.org/article/S0190-9622(17)32051-0/fulltext.

UMBILICAL GRANULOMA

This common cherry-like swelling on a new baby's umbilical stump was previously treated with topical silver nitrate. Concerns about chemical burns with this treatment have led to trials using home treatment with salt:

- Apply enough table salt to cover the granuloma surface
- Cover the area with a gauze swab and keep it in place for 10–30 minutes
- Clean the site using a clean gauze swab soaked in warm water
- Repeat the procedure twice a day for 5 days

Reference

Al Saleh, A. 2016. Therapeutic effect of common salt on umbilical granuloma in infants. *Int J Med Sci Public Health*; 5(5): 911–915. www.ejmanager.com/mnstemps/67/67-1452639453.pdf. doi: 10.5455/ijmsph.2016.07012016312.

ACNE VULGARIS

A chronic condition affecting the hair follicles and sebaceous glands of the face, back and chest, usually starting around puberty.

History
- Distribution
- Previous treatments and results
- Psychological impact
- Taking an oral contraceptive?
- Pregnant, or planning a pregnancy?
- Is it leaving scarring?

Examination
- Mild acne: blackheads (open comedones) and whiteheads (closed comedones)
- Moderate acne: inflamed papules and pustules
- Severe acne: pustules, nodules, scarring and pigmentation

Self-care
- There are many myths about acne – it is not infectious or caused by poor hygiene. Greasy food does not affect it, and sunlight does not improve it
- There is current interest in whether a diet low in refined sugar may be beneficial, but there is no reason to avoid chocolate
- Treatment does not heal existing lesions but prevents new ones, so it may take at least 8 weeks to be visibly effective
- Wash with soap and lukewarm water, just twice daily
- Do not scrub or pick at the skin
- Do not use exfoliants
- Avoid cosmetics as much as possible and remove them completely at night
- If skin is dry, use a water-based emollient
- Mild acne should first be treated with OTC preparations, unless there are exceptional circumstances
- Benzoyl peroxide[C] is the OTC treatment with the best evidence of effectiveness. Unfortunately, only 4% or 5% strengths are currently available, which some people find too irritating. If this is the case, using the treatment just once daily, or even on alternate days only, may help
- See the British Association of Dermatologists' website acnesupport.org.uk for more information

Prescription

- For mild acne with oily skin, if benzoyl peroxide[C] OTC has been tried for 3 months without adequate effect, adapalene[PC] may be prescribed. Women should be counselled regarding the need for contraception with topical retinoids like adapalene[PC] because of the teratogenic risk
- If this causes irritation, offer azelaic acid[C] (but can bleach dark skin)
- If above treatment fails or acne is inflamed, offer combination gel, for example, benzoyl peroxide[C] with adapalene[PC] (Epiduo®[PC]). This is preferred to using combinations including topical antibiotics due to increasing antibiotic resistance
- Consider a combined oral contraceptive, particularly if acne confined to lower face and jaw. This should only be prescribed by a clinician with a family planning qualification. Co-cyprindiol[PBC] is licensed for moderate-to-severe acne not responding to topical treatment or oral antibiotics. It carries a higher venous thromboembolism (VTE) risk than standard combined oral contraceptives (at least double) and should be stopped once the acne has been clear for 3–4 months
- Antibiotic resistance is an increasing problem
- Consider doxycycline[PBC] if topical treatment fails, or if acne is moderate or severe. It has the advantage of a once-daily dosage and can be taken with food. Lymecycline[PBC] appears in some local antimicrobial formularies; it is currently more expensive than doxycycline[PBC]. There is insufficient evidence to support any one tetracycline over another, but minocycline is best avoided because of its higher risk of adverse reactions. **Tetracyclines cannot be used in pregnancy**, and any woman of fertile age requires contraception if using this treatment. Although licensed from the age of 12, most clinicians reserve tetracyclines for older teenagers as they are deposited in growing bones and teeth
- Oral antibiotics should be combined with a topical retinoid (adapalene[PC]) or benzoyl peroxide[C] to limit resistance
- Topical and oral antibiotics should not be used simultaneously
- Refer people with severe acne to Dermatology – and while waiting, initiate treatment with oral antibiotic and topical benzoyl peroxide[C] and adapalene[PC]

Directions and doses for adults

- Apply topical treatments after washing
- Apply benzoyl peroxide[C] once or twice daily
- Apply adapalene[PC] thinly in the evening
- Apply azelaic acid[C] twice daily
- Apply Epiduo®[PC] thinly in the evening
- Doxycycline[PBC] 100 mg once daily
- Lymecycline[PBC] 408 mg twice daily

References

Arowojolu, A.O., Gallo, M.F., Lopez, L.M., and Grimes, D.A. 2012. Combined oral contraceptive pills for treatment of acne. *Cochrane Database Syst Rev*; (7): Art. No.: CD004425. doi: 10.1002/14651858.CD004425.pub6.

Bienenfeld, A., Nagler, A.R., and Orlow, S.J. 2017. Oral antibacterial therapy for acne vulgaris: An evidence-based review. *Am J Clin Dermatol*; 18(4): 469–490. https://link.springer.com/article/10.1007%2Fs40257-017-0267-z. doi: 10.1007/s40257-017-0267-z.

Dawson, A.L., and Dellavalle, R.P. 2013. Acne vulgaris. *BMJ*; 346: f2634. www.bmj.com/content/346/bmj.f2634. doi: 10.1136/bmj.f2634.

Fiedler, F., Stangl, G.I., Fiedler, E., and Taube. K. 2017. Acne and nutrition: A systematic review. *Acta Derm Venereol*; 97: 7–9. www.ingentaconnect.com/contentone/mjl/adv/2017/00000097/00000001/art00003?crawler=true&mimetype=application/pdf.

Magin, P., Pond, D., Smith, W., and Watson, A. 2005. A systematic review of the evidence for 'myths and misconceptions' in acne management: Diet, face-washing and sunlight. *Fam Pract*; 22(1): 62–70. https://academic.oup.com/fampra/article-lookup/doi/10.1093/fampra/cmh715. doi: 10.1093/fampra/cmh715.

Nast, A., Dréno, B., Bettoli, V., Bukvic Mokos, Z., Degitz, K., Dressler, C., Finlay, A.Y. et al. European evidence-based (S3) guideline for the treatment of acne – update 2016 – short version. *J Eur Acad Dermatol Venereol*; 30: 1261–1268. doi:10.1111/jdv.13776.

Simonart, T., Dramaix, M., and De Maertelaer, V. 2008. Efficacy of tetracyclines in the treatment of acne vulgaris: A review. *Br J Dermatol*; 158(2): 208–216. http://onlinelibrary.wiley.com/doi/10.1111/j.1365-2133.2007.08286.x/abstract. doi: 10.1111/j.1365-2133.2007.08286.

Walsh, T.R., Efthimiou, J., and Dréno, B. 2016. Systematic review of antibiotic resistance in acne: An increasing topical and oral threat. *Lancet Infect Dis*; 16(3): e23–e33. *The benefit-to-risk ratio of long-term antibiotic use should be carefully considered and, in particular, use alone avoided where possible.*

CHAPTER 9

Abdomen

ABDOMINAL PAIN

History

- Site and radiation
- Duration
- Intermittent/continuous
- Character: stabbing/dull/colicky
- Previous episodes (diagnosis and outcome)
- Previous abdominal surgery
- Date of last menstrual period (LMP)/vaginal discharge or bleeding/contraception
- Associated features:
    - Fever
    - Constipation/diarrhoea/blood or mucus in stool
    - Vomiting/nausea/loss of appetite
    - Dysuria/frequency/urgency
    - Pain in testicles or groin
    - Upper respiratory tract infection in children (may cause abdominal pain due to enlarged lymph nodes)
- Over-the-counter (OTC) preparations tried
- 🚩 Possibility of pregnancy
- 🚩 Does coughing exacerbate pain?

Examination

- Temperature and pulse rate
- Blood pressure (in adults) and capillary refill time (in children) if unwell or any suspicious of dehydration
- Examine abdomen
    - Confirm site of pain
    - Record site of any tenderness or guarding
    - Check for masses (especially palpable bladder) or distension
    - Check groins for any swellings
    - Check loins for tenderness
- In children, examine tonsils

Tests

- Consider testing urine for protein/blood/glucose/nitrite/pregnancy
- Consider sending midstream urine (MSU) for culture if urinary tract infection (UTI) suspected (unless simple cystitis)
- Consider sending stool sample if food poisoning suspected (see section on Diarrhoea and Vomiting)

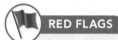

RED FLAGS

- If you are unable to make a firm diagnosis of dyspepsia, UTI or gastroenteritis (*many possible causes; refer to senior clinician*)
- Positive pregnancy test (*ectopic pregnancy may cause severe lower abdominal pain, usually one-sided, in a woman whose period is late or just due. She may not have vaginal bleeding. Refer to Gynaecology same-day*)
- Severe pain causing difficulty climbing on to examination couch, or exacerbated by coughing (*suggests peritonitis; admit under Surgical urgently*)
- Guarding/rigid abdomen (*suggests peritonitis; admit under Surgical urgently*)
- Enlarged bladder with inability to pass urine despite strong urge (*urinary retention; refer to Urology same-day*)
- Pain or swelling in testicles or groin (*possible torsion, infection or hernia; refer urgently to appropriate speciality*)

GASTROENTEROLOGY

1. Dyspepsia/indigestion
2. Diarrhoea and vomiting
3. Constipation
4. Anal problems
5. Threadworms

DYSPEPSIA/INDIGESTION

History

- What does the patient mean by the words they use (like heartburn or reflux)?
- Site of pain – dyspepsia typically presents with central epigastric pain, while upper right-sided pain suggests gallstones
- Feeling of fullness/belching
- Symptoms suggesting reflux (retrosternal pain, tasting acid in the mouth, worse when laying down, sore throat, dry cough)
- Vomiting/nausea/loss of appetite
- Relationship to eating
- Diet (e.g. irregular meals, large meals at night, fatty foods, excessive citrus fruit juices can all cause digestive symptoms)
- Psychosocial stress
- Smoking and alcohol consumption
- Taking medicines which increase risk of gastrointestinal (GI) bleed, for example, anticoagulants, antiplatelet drugs (e.g. aspirin, clopidogrel), non-steroidal anti-inflammatory drugs (NSAIDs), prednisolone, selective serotonin reuptake inhibitors, spironolactone
- Previous episodes, how treated
- Over-the-counter (OTC) preparations tried
- ⚑ Difficulty swallowing
- ⚑ Worse on exercise
- ⚑ Unexplained weight loss
- ⚑ Change in bowel habit
- ⚑ Vomiting of 'coffee-grounds' or dark, tarry stools (melaena)

Examination

- Examine abdomen
- Confirm site of pain
- Check for abnormal swellings or tenderness
- If any suspicion of GI bleed, check pulse rate and blood pressure

Tests

- Public Health England recommends arranging *Helicobacter pylori* (*H. pylori*) testing before prescribing a proton pump inhibitor (PPI) in older people or those from North Africa
  - *H. pylori* testing is unreliable if patient has taken a PPI in previous 2 weeks or antibiotic in previous 4 weeks. If taking a PPI, they will need a 2-week washout period before testing
  - The evidence about ranitidine is unclear, but it probably only needs to be stopped 48 hours before testing, so people taking a PPI can be switched to this if testing for *H. pylori* is required and they cannot cope without medication
  - Antacids can be continued (apart from preparations containing bismuth like Pepto-Bismol® which need to be stopped 2 weeks before testing)
- Consider full blood count (FBC), erythrocyte sedimentation rate (ESR), liver function tests (LFTs) and anti-tissue transglutaminase (anti-TTG)

Self-care

- If overweight, try to lose weight
- If smoker, consider quitting or cutting down
- Reduce alcohol intake
- Avoid any identified triggers such as fatty foods
- Stop NSAIDs, if possible
- If taking aspirin or other gastric irritant medicines, see General Practitioner (GP) to discuss alternatives
- For mild symptoms, try antacids; Mucogel®CI or Gaviscon Advance®CI (both OTC)
- Some PPIs can be bought OTC but should not be used long-term

Prescription

- NHS England has issued guidance advising CCGs against routinely prescribing medicines for indigestion. If there are no concerning features, diet and lifestyle changes and OTC antacids should be tried first, as long as this is clinically appropriate. If a prescription is necessary (perhaps because self-management has not been effective or there are exceptional circumstances), then prescribe omeprazoleQ for 1 month (20 mg daily for adults) and arrange review appointment

RED FLAGS

- Discomfort related to exercise (*may be angina; refer to Medical or rapid access chest pain clinic*)
- On anticoagulant (*at high risk of GI bleed; needs urgent investigation*)
- Difficulty in swallowing (*possible oesophageal cancer; 2-week wait Gastroenterology referral*)
- 'Coffee-ground' or bloodstained vomit or black, tarry stools (*GI bleed; admit under Medical*)
- Aged 40 and over with unexplained weight loss and abdominal pain (*possible bowel cancer; 2-week wait Gastroenterology referral*)
- Aged over 55 with unexplained significant weight loss (*possible gastric cancer; 2-week wait Gastroenterology referral*)

References

NICE NG12. 2017. Suspected cancer: recognition and referral. www.nice.org.uk/guidance/ng12.
Public Health England. 2017. Test and treat for Helicobacter pylori (HP) in dyspepsia. www.gov.uk/government/publications/helicobacter-pylori-diagnosis-and-treatment.

DIARRHOEA AND VOMITING

Viruses cause gastroenteritis much more often than food poisoning; rotavirus and adenovirus are common in children, norovirus in adults. Diarrhoea is the main symptom.

History

- Duration
- Severity: number of episodes in last 24 hours, stool consistency

- Fever
- Fluid balance and urine output (how often are they passing urine)
- Contacts with similar symptoms, especially if they started on the same day
- Suspect foods (undercooked or out-of-date)
- Recent foreign travel or farm visit
- Occupation – food handler/carer/health professional
- Sorbitol (in diet foods, chewing gum–may cause diarrhoea)
- Reptile at home (risk of salmonella infection from handling reptiles)
- Relevant medication that may have caused the symptoms, for example, broad-spectrum antibiotics or laxatives, metformin, colchicine, orlistat
- Taking PPIs (increased risk of *Clostridium difficile* infection)
- Any medications that may be affected by the illness, for example, prednisolone, warfarin, anti-epileptic drugs, angiotensin-converting enzyme (ACE) inhibitors, combined oral contraceptives, gastro-resistant/enteric-coated drugs
- ⚑ Preceding constipation
- ⚑ Blood (red, brown or black) in stool/vomit
- ⚑ Hospital admission in previous 8 weeks
- ⚑ Broad-spectrum antibiotics in previous 8 weeks
- ⚑ Previous bowel disease or gastric bypass
- ⚑ Immunosuppressed
- ⚑ Possibility of pregnancy

Examination

- Temperature
- Dehydration:
  - Lethargy
  - Sunken fontanelle in children under 2 years
  - Dry tongue/mouth
  - Dry skin not reshaping after a soft pinch
  - Sunken eyes
- Pulse rate
- Blood pressure in adults/capillary refill time in children
- Abdominal examination, looking for rigidity or guarding
- Consider rectal examination if overflow suspected (see Red Flags)

Test

- Stool culture if motions are still liquid and:
  - Suspected food poisoning
  - Febrile/systemically unwell
  - Blood or pus in stool
  - Immunosuppressed
  - Recent broad-spectrum antibiotic therapy (also request *C. difficile* test)
  - Recent hospital admission (also request *C. difficile* test)
  - Recent travel to tropical area (also request ova, cysts and parasites)
  - Duration more than 7 days
- Consider stool culture if:
  - Food handler/carer/healthcare staff/in contact with vulnerable people (check with Health Protection Team [HPT])
  - Pregnant

- On proton pump inhibitor (PPI)

(Recommended method: ask patient to collect 5 ml sample from clingfilm-lined container. Write patient's name on specimen bottle, or affix label, before giving out. Less than 5% of samples will identify a bacterial cause.)

- Also check urine dipstick and MSU in children under 5 years with persistent or recurrent diarrhoea or vomiting (see Urology section)

Self-care

- Give reassurance: rarely serious in primary care and usually has viral cause
- Do not return to work/school/day care until free of symptoms for 48 hours
- If cryptosporidium is diagnosed, do not swim in public pools for 2 weeks
- Dehydration is rare over 6 months of age (explain warning signs)
- Give worsening advice and make sure the patient is aware of the symptoms of dehydration. Gastroenteritis normally resolves in 5–7 days
- Eating and drinking:
  - Sip extra fluids, for example, 200 ml for each loose stool in adults
  - Avoid orange juice and fizzy drinks, but isotonic still sports drinks are a good option. Gatorade contains potassium, which replaces losses from both the gut and the kidneys (renal excretion of potassium increases after vomiting to maintain acid-base balance)
  - Advise against replacing fluid losses with plain water or home-manufactured salt solution
  - Supplement with purchased oral rehydration solution (ORS) if:
    - Child under 2 years, especially if under 6 months or premature
    - Diarrhoea > 5 times in 24 hours
    - Vomiting > 2 times in 24 hours
    - Frail, malnourished or elderly
  - Half-strength apple juice has recently shown to be preferable to ORS in children with mild gastroenteritis (Freedman et al., 2016)
  - Fasting is not recommended. A normal diet should be resumed as soon as symptoms permit. Warn about the gastro-colic reflex (often mistaken as food 'going straight through' the patient)
  - Babies should continue normal feeds. There is no need to restrict dairy products unless diarrhoea is prolonged and lactose intolerance is suspected (Box 9.1)
- Hygiene advice to patient
  - Take care when washing hands after using toilet/changing nappy
  - Remember to use the clean hand (i.e. not the one which has been used for wiping) to flush the toilet and turn on the taps
  - Close the toilet lid before you flush
  - Toilet seats, handles, taps and toilet door handles should be cleaned at least daily with hot water and detergent. Also use disinfectant or bleach to clean toilets
  - Soiled clothing should be washed separately at the highest temperature it will tolerate
- Self-care with OTC medication
  - Paracetamol may be taken for stomach cramps
  - Avoid NSAIDs (gut irritants)
  - Probiotics such as *Lactobacillus acidophilus* may be helpful, especially in diarrhoea following broad-spectrum antibiotics. They should not be taken by immunosuppressed patients
  - Loperamide[PCQ] may be taken by adults if diarrhoea is disabling, but not to enable return to work. Avoid if there is fever, blood in the stool, *C. difficile* or severe malaise. 'The body has evolved for our survival, and not for our comfort'
  - Buccal prochlorperazine[PBCQ] may be helpful to stop vomiting in adults who are at risk of dehydration or need to take essential medication, but carries the rare risk, particularly in young adults, of an oculogyric crisis (adult dose 3–6 mg up to twice daily, tablets to be placed high between upper lip and gum and left to dissolve)

> **BOX 9.1 LACTOSE INTOLERANCE**
>
> Occasionally, after a bout of gastroenteritis, small children may develop a temporary inability to digest lactose, which may delay the resolution of their diarrhoea. If this is suspected, suggest using lactose-free milk (e.g. SMA LF®) and a lactose-free diet for up to 6 weeks.

Prescription (none for most patients)

- Antibiotics should not be used unless a specific bacterial/protozoal cause has been identified through culture, and a specific treatment is indicated

Action

- Advise about medication, for example, combined oral contraceptive (COC)
- Consider stopping PPI, which reduces the natural defences against GI infection
- If patient is at risk of dehydration or low blood pressure, advise temporarily stopping the DAMN drugs to reduce the risk of acute kidney injury (AKI):
  - **D**iuretics/**D**igoxin
  - **A**ngiotensin converting enzyme (ACE) inhibitors/**A**ngiotensin receptor blockers (ARB)
  - **M**etformin/**M**ethotrexate
  - **N**SAIDs
- Notify HPT immediately, and inform patient, if:
  - Food poisoning suspected because of history
  - Blood or pus in stool
  - Bacterial or protozoal infection confirmed by culture

RED FLAGS

- Dehydration (*admit under Medical/Paediatrics*)
- Severe illness (*consider sepsis; admit under Medical/Paediatrics*)
- Immunosuppressed (*high risk for serious illness or unusual microbial cause; may need admission*)
- Taking oral prednisolone or dexamethasone (*at risk of adrenal crisis; consider IM/IV hydrocortisone and/or admission for IV fluids*)
- Taking other essential medication, e.g. anticonvulsants or medicines for Parkinson's Disease (*discuss with senior colleague*)
- Diabetes (*will need careful blood glucose [BG] monitoring and adjustment of medication*)
- Bowel disease, for example, ulcerative colitis, Crohn's disease, diverticular disease (*seek specialist advice; e.g. IBD nurse*)
- Green vomit (*suggests obstruction; admit under Surgical*)
- Significant blood loss: red or brown vomit/red or black stools (*likely GI bleed; admit under Medical*)
- Early pregnancy (*ectopic pregnancy may cause vomiting and diarrhoea without vaginal bleeding; refer to Gynaecology urgently*)
- Abdominal rigidity or guarding (*admit under Surgical*)
- Previous constipation (*possible faecal impaction and overflow; arrange rectal examination*)
- Hyperventilation and/or breath that smells of over-ripe fruit (mild) / nail polish remover (severe) (*possible diabetic ketoacidosis; check blood glucose and urine ketones*)

References

Allen, S.J., Martinez, E.G., Gregorio, G.V., and Dans, L.F. 2010. Probiotics for treating acute infectious diarrhoea. *Cochrane Database Syst Rev*; (11). Art. No.: CD003048. doi: 10.1002/14651858.CD003048.pub3. *Probiotics appear to be safe and have clear beneficial effects in shortening the duration and reducing stool frequency in acute infectious diarrhea.*

Freedman, S.B., Willan, A.R., Boutis, K., and Schuh, S. 2016. Effect of dilute apple juice and preferred fluids vs electrolyte maintenance solution on treatment failure among children with mild gastroenteritis. A randomized clinical trial. *JAMA*; 315(18):1966–1974. doi: 10.1001/jama.2016.5352

Goldenberg, J.Z., Lytvyn, L., Steurich, J., Parkin, P., Mahant, S., and Johnston, B.C. 2015. Probiotics for the prevention of pediatric antibiotic-associated diarrhea. *Cochrane Database Syst Rev*; (12). Art. No.: CD004827. doi: 10.1002/14651858.CD004827.pub4. *Moderate quality evidence suggests a protective effect of probiotics in preventing AAD with a NNT of 10.*

Goldenberg, J.Z., Ma, S.S.Y., Saxton, J.D., Martzen, M.R., Vandvik, P.O., Thorlund, K., Guyatt, G.H., and Johnston, B.C. 2013. Probiotics for the prevention of Clostridium difficile-associated diarrhea in adults and children. *Cochrane Database Syst Rev*; Issue (5). Art. No.: CD006095. doi: 10.1002/14651858.CD006095.pub3. *Moderate quality evidence suggests that probiotics are both safe and effective for preventing Clostridium difficile-associated diarrhoea.*

Masukume, G. 2011. Nausea, vomiting and deaths from ectopic pregnancy (letter). *BMJ*; 343:d4389. doi: 10.1136/bmj.d4389. *More than a third of women who have died because of ectopic pregnancy in the United Kingdom since 1997 had nausea, vomiting and diarrhoea but no vaginal bleeding.*

NICE CG84. 2009. Diarrhoea and vomiting caused by gastroenteritis in children under 5. www.nice.org.uk/guidance/CG84.

Public Health England. 2013. UK standards for microbiology investigations gastroenteritis and diarrhoea. www.gov.uk/government/uploads/system/uploads/attachment_data/file/344110/S_7i1.pdf. *Stool sampling recommendations.*

Think Kidneys. 2017. www.thinkkidneys.nhs.uk/aki/resources/primary-care. *Advice on avoiding and managing acute kidney injury.*

World Gastroenterology Organisation. 2012. Acute diarrhea in adults and children: A global perspective. www.worldgastroenterology.org/guidelines/global-guidelines/acute-diarrhea.

CONSTIPATION

Though this is strictly defined by NICE as 'defecation that is unsatisfactory because of infrequent stools (fewer than three times a week), difficult stool passage or seeming incomplete', it is arguably better to define constipation as a change from a person's usual bowel pattern towards less frequent stools.

History

- Duration; habitual
- How often bowels opened
- Consistency of motion
- Difficulty passing stools/straining
- Abdominal pain
- Vomiting
- Fluid intake
- Amount of exercise
- Previous abdominal operations
- Medication (e.g. opioids, iron, PPIs, anti-muscarinics [e.g. oxybutynin])
- 🚩 Blood in stool, on toilet paper or in toilet pan (not always a red flag – see box below for details)
- 🚩 Unintentional weight loss

Examination

- Examine abdomen
- Consider rectal examination if unclear whether the patient has faecal impaction/loading

Self-care

- Stop any constipating medicine, if possible
- Adequate fluid intake (2 l per day, including that from food)
- Increase exercise
- Consider resting feet on a step while sitting on the toilet, leaning forward with elbows on knees to relax the puborectalis muscle
- Increase intake of whole grains, apples, apricots, prunes and dried fruit. Dried fruits are high in sorbitol, a natural laxative
- Try Beverley-Travis natural laxative mixture: take 1 cup each of raisins, pitted prunes, prune concentrate, dried figs, dates and currants. Combine contents together in grinder or blender to a thickened consistency. Store in refrigerator. Dose: 2 tablespoons twice a day. Increase or decrease dose according to consistency and frequency of bowel movements
- Bulk-forming laxatives such as ispaghula husk are first line in adults (one sachet twice daily, dose to be given in water preferably after meals, morning and evening) except for constipation caused by opioids (see below). An adequate fluid intake is important

Laxatives

- In children, do not use dietary measures alone. Prescribe macrogols[CP] (*unlicensed for children under 2 years*). See NICE guideline CG99 for more information

- NHS England has issued guidance to CCGs advising against prescriptions to treat short term, infrequent constipation caused by changes in lifestyle or diet. In adults, this should be managed through self-care and OTC laxatives if necessary. This guidance does not apply to longer-term constipation or symptoms relating to organic disease or medication side effects

- If stools remain hard, change to macrogols[CP] (adult dose: one to three sachets daily in divided doses usually for up to 2 weeks; maintenance one to two sachets daily). Clinical Knowledge Summaries (CKS) does not recommend their use in pregnancy because of the theoretical risk of electrolyte imbalance caused by osmosis, although there have been no reported problems

- If stools are soft but still difficult to pass, add a stimulant laxative such as senna[C] (adult dose: 7.5–15 mg at bedtime, increased if necessary up to 30 mg) or bisacodyl[C] (adult dose: 5–10 mg at night, increased if necessary up to 20 mg)

- Treatment may need to continue for several weeks

- Adults with faecal loading need high-dose oral macrogol[CP] (initially four sachets daily on first day, then increased in steps of two sachets daily, total daily dose to be drunk within a 6-hour period. After disimpaction, switch to maintenance laxative therapy if required; maximum eight sachets per day) or, for faster relief, glycerol suppositories (4 g for adults) or an enema

- For opioid-induced constipation, use docusate orally (up to 500 mg daily in divided doses for adults, adjusted according to response) *or* a combination of an osmotic laxative (e.g. lactulose 15 ml twice daily for adults, adjusted according to response) to soften the stool and a stimulant laxative (e.g. adult dose: senna[C] 7.5–15 mg at bedtime, increased if necessary up to 30 mg)

RED FLAGS

- 2-week wait referral for suspected lower GI cancer if:
  - Age ≥40 with unexplained weight loss and abdominal pain
  - Aged <50 with rectal bleeding and any of the following:
    - Abdominal pain
    - Altered bowel habit
    - Weight loss
    - Iron-deficiency anaemia
  - Aged ≥50 with unexplained rectal bleeding
  - Aged ≥60 with alteration in bowel habit or iron-deficiency anaemia
- Constipation associated with vomiting, distension and/or previous abdominal surgery (*possible bowel obstruction; admit under Surgical*)
- Mass in abdomen other than a loaded descending colon (*2-week wait referral for suspected lower GI cancer*)
- In child, symptoms from first few weeks of life (*possible Hirschsprung's disease; refer to Paediatrics*)

References

Hale, E.M., Smith, E., St. James, J., and Wojner-Alexandrov, A.W. 2007. Pilot study of the feasibility and effectiveness of a natural laxative mixture. *Geriatr Nurs*; 28(2):104–111. www.gnjournal.com/article/S0197-4572(06)00291-6/fulltext. doi: 10.1016/j.gerinurse.2006.10.002. *Evidence for the Beverley-Travis mixture*.

NICE CG99. 2017. Constipation in children and young people: Diagnosis and management. www.nice.org.uk/guidance/cg99.

NICE CKS. 2017. Constipation. cks.nice.org.uk/constipation.

NICE NG12. 2017. Suspected cancer: Recognition and referral. www.nice.org.uk/guidance/ng12.

ANAL PROBLEMS

Haemorrhoids ('piles')

These are distended venous cushions inside the anal canal, which have a similar appearance to varicose veins. They may prolapse ('come down') on straining, when they may be visible as soft, purple grape-like swellings protruding from the anus. External haemorrhoids may cause bleeding, itching or discomfort. Internal haemorrhoids have no pain and may cause no symptoms apart from bleeding.

Thrombosed external pile

This is caused by a sudden swelling of a small blood vessel near the anus (usually after straining). The blood stretches the sensitive skin, which is very painful. It will gradually disperse, but if the patient presents early, it is possible for someone with adequate surgical experience to incise it and relieve pain by releasing the blood clot.

Anal fissure

A split or an ulcer in the anal skin, previously thought to be caused by passing a large, hard stool but now considered to be an ischaemic ulcer. This is a common cause of pain and bleeding on defaecation. Most will heal within 6 weeks, provided that the stools remain soft.

History

- Bleeding on defaecation:
  - How much blood and where is it seen? i.e., in toilet pan/on paper only
  - Bright red/dark red
- Pain on defaecation (suggests anal fissure, but suspect threadworms in children)
- Itch (suspect threadworms in children)
- Swelling near anus/swelling appearing on straining (may be felt when wiping)
- Background of constipation
- Treatments tried already

Examination (may be normal if haemorrhoids are internal)

- Any visible swelling on the perianal skin (thrombosed external piles) or protruding through the anus (prolapsed internal piles)
- Any split in perianal skin (anal fissure)
- Threadworms may be seen

Self-care

- Avoid straining
- High-fibre diet (see Self Care in Constipation section)
- Drink 2 l of fluid daily
- Use moist wipes, then pat area dry
- If the pain of thrombosed piles or anal fissure is severe, relief may be obtained by sitting in a warm bath or applying a bag of frozen peas to the area (which will mould to the right shape)
- Consider ispaghula husk
- Anusol[C] (OTC) ointment and/or suppositories may give symptomatic relief (use twice daily, morning and night, plus additional doses after a bowel movement)

Action

- NHS England have released guidance to CCGs advising against prescribing routinely for haemorrhoids. This would not seem applicable to thrombosed external piles where the considerable pain may warrant medication which is not available OTC
- Preparations containing local anaesthetic may give better pain relief but could cause sensitisation if used for more than a few days. Preparations containing topical steroids may reduce inflammation but can exacerbate any local infection. Prescribe hydrocortisone with lidocaine[CP] ointment (use several times daily) or spray (use up to three times daily) if pain is severe (for no more than 7 days)

RED FLAGS

- Severe pain from external thrombosed piles or prolapsed internal piles (*admit under Surgical for excision*)
- Painless rectal bleeding with dark blood (*may come from a carcinoma high inside the bowel*). Therefore, *2-week wait for suspected lower GI cancer if:*
  - Aged <50 with rectal bleeding and any of the following:
    - Abdominal pain
    - Altered bowel habit
    - Weight loss
    - Iron-deficiency anaemia
  - Aged ≥50 with unexplained rectal bleeding

THREADWORMS

History

- Children most commonly affected
- Perianal irritation
- Anal pain at night
- Sometimes vaginal itching
- Worms may be seen – like white cotton threads – on skin or in stool

Examination

- Examine the affected area for worms/trauma

Test

No testing is necessary unless the diagnosis is in doubt:

- Your microbiology laboratory may supply a 'pinworm kit' containing a sticky slide. This should be applied to the anus first thing in the morning to pick up the eggs

Self-care

- An appointment is not necessary if the parent is sure of the diagnosis
- Explain that adult threadworms live for only 6 weeks – their eggs must be transferred to the mouth and swallowed for the infection to continue
- No need to exclude from school/day care
- Hygienic measures are necessary:
  - Change and launder bed linen, underwear, cuddly toys and night clothes
  - Vacuum bedroom carpet and mattress and damp-dust the bathroom
  - Cut fingernails short, and consider cotton gloves at night
  - Do not put fingers in the mouth
  - Wash hands and scrub nails before each meal and after going to the toilet
  - For 2 weeks:
    - Wear close-fitting underpants/knickers in bed and change them every morning
    - Bathe or shower the perianal area in early morning to remove eggs laid during the night, and wet-wipe the area at 3 hourly intervals, if possible

Treatment

- Mebendazole[PBC] (OTC) 100 mg single dose for adults (unless pregnant or breastfeeding) and children over 2 years old. A second dose may be needed two weeks later. Unless there are exceptional circumstances, this medicine should be obtained OTC rather than prescribed. However, children aged 6 months to 2 years will need a prescription (*unlicensed indication*).
- Treat all household members simultaneously
- If aged under six months, pregnant or breastfeeding, hygiene methods alone should be used

References

NICE CKS. 2016a. Anal fissure. cks.nice.org.uk/anal-fissure.
NICE CKS. 2016b. Haemorrhoids. cks.nice.org.uk/haemorrhoids.
NICE NG12. 2017. Suspected cancer: recognition and referral. www.nice.org.uk/guidance/ng12.
NICE CKS. 2018. Threadworm. cks.nice.org.uk/threadworm.

UROLOGY

1. Cystitis
2. Pyelonephritis
3. Balanitis

CYSTITIS (LOWER URINARY TRACT INFECTION)

History
- Duration
- Dysuria
- Urgency
- Frequency and nocturia
- Suprapubic discomfort/pain
- Cloudy, red-brown or offensive urine (if the urine is not cloudy, there is only a 3% chance of UTI [SIGN 2012])
- Incontinence/bedwetting
- Vaginal discharge
- Sexual history (see the start of Chapter 10)
- Symptoms associated with intercourse
- Possibility of pregnancy
- Previous history of kidney disease
- In men, symptoms of urinary obstruction (hesitancy, straining, poor stream)
- 🚩 In men, symptoms of prostatitis (fever, perineal pain)
- 🚩 Fever

Examination
- Temperature
- Pulse rate
- Check loins for tenderness
- In children, men or anyone with suspected pyelonephritis, examine abdomen and check for palpable bladder
- In a menopausal woman with recurrent symptoms, offer examination for atrophic vaginitis
- In small boys, check the penis for redness (see section on Balanitis)

Tests
- **Urinalysis is not necessary in 'simple cystitis'** (lower UTI in a non-pregnant, low-risk adult woman). Consider urinalysis for blood/leucocyte esterase/nitrite only if the diagnosis of lower UTI is in doubt
- Urinalysis and MSU before starting treatment in:
  - Children – a clean-catch sample should be collected in a sterile container, for example, a universal container or gallipot. Clean, but non-sterile containers, can be used at home if no sterile container is available, but they are best lined with clingfilm to reduce contamination. For young girls who can use a toilet, it may make it easier to collect the sample if they sit facing the cistern (Kaufman et al., 2017). In babies, wiping the abdomen repeatedly with a cold wet solution encourages urination ('Quick Wee Method')
  - Men
  - Pregnant women
  - Immunosuppressed
  - Recurrent infections
  - Previous treatment failure
- A positive nitrite test is 90% diagnostic of infection (Public Health England 2017a), but a negative result for all three indicators does not exclude infection
- Urinalysis strips are not sterile and contain many different chemicals. If you are intending to send the sample to the laboratory, it should not be contaminated with a dipstick
- Many urinalysis strips are unsuitable for use with the red-top bottles containing boric acid; false negatives may occur. The only brand which we have been assured is compatible is Medi-Test Combi 8®
- Arrange follow-up MSU after treatment in pregnant women or repeat the dipstick if haematuria is present (to check that the infection/haematuria has resolved)

- Consider chlamydia test if suggested by sexual history, a change in vaginal discharge, pain or bleeding during or after sexual intercourse
- Asymptomatic bacteriuria is common in older people (25% of women and 10% of men over 65). It should not be treated (even if found at a pre-op assessment; see Mayne et al., 2016)
- Catheterised patients' bladders are often colonised by bacteria; there is no evidence that treatment with antibiotics will benefit them, unless they have at least one of the following: fever, new costovertebral tenderness, rigors or new-onset delirium

Self-care

- Adequate fluid intake
- Excessive fluid intake may increase the amount of dysuria in 24 hours; there is no evidence that it speeds recovery
- Avoid OTC remedies such as Cymalon® or CanesOasis®; they are ineffective (O'Kane et al., 2016) and may interfere with antibiotic treatment
- Cranberry extract is also ineffective for the *treatment* of UTI, and interacts with warfarin
- If cystitis recurs despite self-care, consider *prophylactic* cranberry products (Fu et al., 2017, Roshdibonab et al., 2017) or D-mannose[P] supplements (Kranjčec et al., 2014).
- If cystitis tends to occur after sexual intercourse, advise emptying bladder immediately after intercourse

Action

- Offer antibiotics for all except minor urinary infections
- Do not wait for the MSU result before starting antibiotics, especially in pregnancy (UTI in early pregnancy increases the risk of miscarriage)
- Advise against excessive fluid intake, as this may impair the adequate concentration of antibiotic in the urinary tract, as well as increasing the number of episodes of dysuria
- Simple cystitis in a non-pregnant woman:
  - Without antibiotics, resolves in 4–9 days
  - With antibiotics, resolves in 3–8 days
  - On average, antibiotics shorten duration by 1 day
- In children, if either nitrite or leucocyte esterase are positive, start antibiotic without waiting for MSU result (NICE 2017)
- Plan to review children and pregnant women by phone when MSU result is available. In pregnant women, arrange a post-treatment MSU
- Growth of $> 10^4$ organisms per ml is now accepted as diagnostic of a UTI. If MSU shows that the organism is resistant to the antibiotic prescribed, check with patient whether their symptoms have resolved. Laboratory sensitivity data do not necessarily reflect what happens to the patient
- Risk factors for increased antibiotic resistance include care home resident, recurrent UTI, hospitalisation for >7d in the last 6 months, unresolving urinary symptoms, recent travel to a country with increased resistance and previous resistant UTI

Antibiotic choice

Before the MSU result is known, choice depends on local sensitivities. Consult local guidelines, or ask your microbiologist about the local resistance pattern. Trimethoprim has high levels of resistance nationally and should not be prescribed if the patient has taken it within the previous three months.

- Simple cystitis, for 3 days:
  - Nitrofurantoin MR[PBC] *or*
  - Trimethoprim[PI] *or*
  - Pivmecillinam[P] *or*
  - Fosfomycin[PC]
- Cystitis in a woman with chronic kidney disease (CKD), abnormal renal tract or immunosuppression: consider extending course to 5–7 days
- Pregnant woman: nitrofurantoin MR[PBC] for 7 days (unless 36 weeks pregnant or more, in which case use cefalexin)
- Men: treat simple cystitis with nitrofurantoin MR[PBC] for 7 days. Note this would not be adequate if there is a suspicion of prostatic involvement (fever, perineal or lower abdominal or back pain, pain on ejaculation, urethral discharge)

- Children: trimethoprim[PI] for 3 days (or cefalexin for 3 days if allergic to trimethoprim). Although nitrofurantoin oral suspension[PB] is recommended by national guidance, the liquid preparation is prohibitively expensive
- Do not use amoxicillin for UTI unless there is an MSU result showing that the organism is sensitive (50% are resistant)

Doses in adults

- Nitrofurantoin MR[PBC] 100 mg twice daily
- Trimethoprim[PI] 200 mg twice daily
- Pivmecillinam[P] 400 mg initially, then 200 mg three times daily
- Cefalexin 500 mg twice daily
- Fosfomycin[PC] 3 g single dose

Prescription warnings

Nitrofurantoin[PBC] may produce neonatal haemolysis if used near term or in breastfeeding if the infant is susceptible. **Trimethoprim**[PI] has serious interactions with methotrexate, azathioprine, ciclosporin, mercaptopurine and tacrolimus, so be aware when prescribing for a patient with a long-term inflammatory condition such as rheumatoid arthritis. Trimethoprim also interacts significantly with phenytoin.
Pivmecillinam[P] is a prodrug of mecillinam, a penicillin, so cannot be used for those allergic to penicillin.

 RED FLAGS

- Aged under three months (*high risk; admit under Paediatrics*)
- Fever (*suspect pyelonephritis or prostatitis: refer to senior colleague*)
- Palpable bladder (*bladder outlet obstruction; refer to Urology for urgent catheterisation*)
- Child or pregnant woman not responding to antibiotics after 48hr (*high risk; review and change antibiotic or refer to senior colleague*)
- A child with confirmed UTI may need *referral for imaging*, particularly if:
  - Aged under 6 months
  - Infected with an organism which is not *Escherichia coli*
  - Three or more episodes of lower UTI
- A man with symptoms of urinary obstruction, e.g. hesitancy, straining, or poor stream (*suggests prostatic problem; refer to senior colleague*)
- Persistent or unexplained haematuria (*possible urological cancer; may require 2-week wait referral*)

References

Delanghe, J., and Speeckaert, M. 2014. Preanalytical requirements of urinalysis. *Biochemia Medica*; 24(1):89–104. www.ncbi.nlm.nih.gov/pmc/articles/PMC3936984/. doi: 10.11613/BM.2014.011. *Boric acid keeps urinary pH below 7, prevents dissolution of pus cells, and is associated with false-negative strip test results (e.g. protein, white blood cells and ketones).*

Fu, Z., Liska, D., Talan, D., and Chung, M., 2017. Cranberry reduces the risk of urinary tract infection recurrence in otherwise healthy women: A systematic review and meta-analysis. *J Nutr*; 147(12):2282–2288.

Kaufman, J., Fitzpatrick, P., Tosif, S., Hopper, S., Donath, S.M., Bryant, P.A., and Babl, F.E. 2017. Faster clean catch urine collection (Quick-Wee method) from infants: Randomised controlled trial. *BMJ*; 357:j1341. doi: 10.1136/bmj.j1341. *Quick-Wee is a simple cutaneous stimulation method that significantly increases the 5-minute voiding and success rate of clean catch urine collection.*

Kranjčec, B., Papeš, D., and Altarac, S. 2014. D-mannose powder for prophylaxis of recurrent urinary tract infections in women: A randomized clinical trial. *World J Urol*; 32:79. doi.org/10.1007/s00345-013-1091-6. *2 g of D-mannose powder in 200 mL of water daily reduced the risk of recurrent UTI (NNT 3) to the same degree as prophylactic nitrofurantoin.*

Mayne, A.I.W., Davies, P.S.E., and Simpson, J.M. 2016. Screening for asymptomatic bacteriuria before total joint arthroplasty. *BMJ*; 354:i3569. doi: 10.1136/bmj.i3569. *Patients with asymptomatic bacteriuria have an increased risk of (joint) infection, but current evidence does not support routine antibiotic treatment before arthroplasty.*

Naber, K.G. 2000. Treatment options for acute uncomplicated cystitis in adults. *J Antimicrob Chemother*; 46(suppl 1):S23–S27. *Antibiotic treatment for 3 days is as effective as longer duration.*

NICE. 2019. Urinary tract infections (lower): Antimicrobial prescribing. Not yet published. www.nice.org.uk/guidance/indevelopment/gid-apg10004.

NICE CG54. 2017. Urinary tract infection in under 16s: Diagnosis and management. www.nice.org.uk/guidance/cg54.

O'Kane, D.B., Dave, S.K., Gore, N., Patel, F., Hoffmann, T.C., Trill, J.L., and Del Mar CB. 2016. Urinary alkalisation for symptomatic uncomplicated urinary tract infection in women. *Cochrane Database Syst Rev*; Issue:(4). Art. No.: CD010745. doi: 10.1002/14651858. CD010745.pub2

Perrotta, C., Aznar, M., Mejia, R., Albert, X., and Ng, C.W. 2008. Oestrogens for preventing recurrent urinary tract infection in postmenopausal women. *Cochrane Database Syst Rev*; Issue:(2). Art. No.: CD005131. doi: 10.1002/14651858.CD005131.pub2. *Based on only two studies comparing vaginal oestrogens to placebo, vaginal oestrogens reduced the number of UTIs in postmenopausal women with recurrent UTI; however, this varied according to the type of oestrogen used and the treatment duration.*

Public Health England. 2017a. Diagnosis of urinary tract infections. Quick reference guide for primary care: For consultation and local adaptation. www.gov.uk/government/publications/urinary-tract-infection-diagnosis.

Public Health England. 2017b. Management and treatment of common infections. www.gov.uk/government/publications/managing-common-infections-guidance-for-primary-care.

Roshdibonab, F., FazlJoo, M., Mohammadbager, S., Torbati, M., Mohammadi, G., Asadloo, M., and Noshad, H., 2017. The role of cranberry in preventing urinary tract infection in children; a systematic review and meta-analysis. *Int J Pediatr*; 5(12):6457–6468.

SIGN 88. 2012 Management of suspected bacterial urinary tract infection in adults: A national clinical guideline. www.sign.ac.uk/sign-88-management-of-suspected-bacterial-urinary-tract-infection-in-adults.html.

PYELONEPHRITIS (UPPER URINARY TRACT INFECTION)

A bacterial infection of the kidney, usually caused by infection spreading up the ureters. It is commoner in children who have vesico-ureteric reflux and in pregnancy, when the ureters are dilated.

History
- There may be symptoms of cystitis (see previous section) – but these can be absent
- Fever/rigors
- Loin pain/suprapubic pain
- Vomiting
- Feeling very unwell/confusion
- In babies: fever/vomiting/poor feeding/diarrhoea

Examination
- Temperature
- Pulse rate
- Blood pressure in adults/capillary refill time in children
- Check loins for tenderness
- Examine abdomen for palpable bladder

Tests
- Urinalysis for blood/leucocyte esterase/nitrites
- MSU before starting treatment

Self-care
- Adequate fluid intake (but not excessive)
- Analgesia – paracetamol
- Worsening advice

Action
- Pyelonephritis is not a minor illness and should only be managed by experienced clinicians
- Consider hospital admission for children and pregnant women
- Prescribe an antibiotic (see section that follows)
- Review after 24 hours, and again when MSU result is available

Antibiotic choice (depends on local sensitivities)

Treat for 7 days with one of the following options:

- Cefalexin (500 mg three times daily), including for use in pregnancy
- Ciprofloxacin^{PCIQ} (500 mg twice daily)
- Co-amoxiclav (500/125 mg three times daily)

See NMIC website for debate on antibiotic choice.

Nitrofurantoin is **not** suitable for treating pyelonephritis because it does not achieve adequate concentration of the antibiotic in the blood or the tissue of the kidney

RED FLAGS

- Sepsis – including low BP, rapid pulse, systemically unwell (*admit under Medical via 999 ambulance*)
- Dehydrated (*if not tolerating oral fluids, may need admission under Medical*)
- Palpable bladder (*admit under Medical*)
- Immunosuppressed (*seek advice from a senior clinician*)
- Diabetes (*will need careful BG monitoring and adjustment of medication*)
- Renal disease (*seek advice from a senior clinician*)
- Pregnant (*admit under Medical*)
- Child (*risk of long-term renal scarring; admit under Paediatrics*)
- Refer routinely, for investigation, if:
  - Male
  - More than two episodes of pyelonephritis
  - MSU shows Proteus infection

References

Harding, M. 2016. Pyelonephritis. patient.info/doctor/pyelonephritis.
NICE CKS. 2013. Pyelonephritis – acute. cks.nice.org.uk/pyelonephritis-acute.

BALANITIS (INFLAMMATION OF THE GLANS PENIS)

This occurs at all ages and may be due to dermatitis, fungal or bacterial infection.

History

- Duration
- Swelling of foreskin
- Discharge
- Itch/odour
- Dysuria
- Consider possibility of diabetes: risk factors (family history, ethnicity, obesity, hypertension) or suggestive symptoms (excessive thirst and polyuria)
- Sexual history (in adults) (see the start of Chapter 10)
- 🚩 Immunosuppressed

Examination

- Gently attempt to retract foreskin in boys aged 3 years and over
- Assess hygiene, look for discharge
- Localised redness/generalised cellulitis

RED FLAGS

- Immunosuppressed/severe symptoms (*refer to Sexual Health*)
- Consider diabetes; this may be the first presentation (*check fasting plasma glucose or HbA1c if appropriate; see Box 8.2 [Checking for Diabetes] in Chapter 8*)

Tests

- Consider taking a swab if severe

Self-care

- Advise gentle cleaning with lukewarm water
- Avoid soap, bubble bath and shower gel
- Do not attempt to pull back the foreskin if it is tight
- If difficulty passing urine because of pain, then advise sitting in bath

Prescription

- Clotrimazole/hydrocortisone cream for 7 days for mild inflammation (apply thinly and evenly, twice daily, and rub in gently)
- If cellulitis is present, flucloxacillin for 7 days (250 mg four times daily in adults) or, if allergic to penicillin, clarithromycin[PIQ] (250 mg twice daily in adults)

References

Imm, N. 2016 Balanitis. patient.info/doctor/balanitis-pro.
NICE CKS. 2015. Balanitis. cks.nice.org.uk/balanitis.

CHAPTER 10

Women's health

TAKING A SEXUAL HISTORY

- Establish rapport first
- Explain that you need to ask some sensitive questions to establish what is wrong
- Last sexual intercourse, partner gender (and age if patient <18 years or vulnerable), sites of exposure, condom use
- Previous sexual partners in the last 12 months
- Previous sexually transmitted infections (STIs)
- Last menstrual period (LMP), contraceptive history
- Establish if there is an impairment of capacity or any safeguarding issues

For more information see the British Association for Sexual Health and HIV guideline: https://shivtoolkit.wordpress.com/worksheets-and-group-activities.

VAGINAL DISCHARGE

The two commonest causes of abnormal vaginal discharge in primary care are bacterial vaginosis (BV) and candida. BV is more common than candida but under-diagnosed, candida is over-diagnosed and over-treated. It is important not to miss a sexually transmitted infection (STI) or pelvic inflammatory disease.

History
- Duration
- Any itch? Any unpleasant odour? Any skin changes?
- Any treatments tried already?
- Recurrent symptoms?
- Is she at increased risk of a sexually transmitted infection (STI)?
    - Age under 25 years
    - Previous STIs
    - Recent new partner
    - More than one sexual partner in past year
    - Partner has symptoms of STI
- Immunosuppressed?
- Symptoms suggesting pelvic inflammatory disease:
    - Abdominal pain/pain during intercourse/dysuria
    - Fever
    - Irregular bleeding/post-coital bleeding/bloodstained or brown discharge
- Vulval pain or blisters (*genital herpes?*)
- Offensive discharge (*retained tampon?*)
- Any other worrying symptoms, e.g. unusual bleeding or pelvic pain?
- Any recent pregnancy or gynaecological procedure (*high risk of sepsis*)?

Examination (see Figure 10.1)

- If systemically unwell, check temperature, pulse rate and blood pressure
- If red flag symptoms are present, digital vaginal and speculum examination is indicated:
  - It may sometimes be preferable for this examination to be performed by the Sexual Health service (where immediate microscopy is available) – discuss the options with the patient, but make sure to avoid undue delay
  - Urgent referral to Gynaecology may be needed in certain situations – see Red Flags box below
  - If there is any possibility of an ectopic pregnancy, internal examination should not be performed in primary care
  - A chaperone should always be offered for intimate examinations
- Painful vesicles are suggestive of genital herpes (*offer oral aciclovir and refer to Sexual Health, but ensure patient is aware that infection may not have come from her current partner*)
- If no red flags are present, then examination is unnecessary, and the patient should be offered pH testing (see below)
- If the diagnosis is uncertain, refer to Sexual Health service for examination

Tests

- Offer vaginal pH testing (which may be done by the patient), and, if accepted, use pH to guide treatment (see Box 10.1):
  - If itch but no offensive odour, pH 4.5 or less: treat for candida
  - If offensive odour but no itch, pH more than 4.5: treat for BV
- High vaginal swabs traditionally have been used to guide the treatment of vaginal discharge, but a national guideline (Lazaro, 2013) states that there is no evidence that they are useful. Their diagnostic yield is poor with over-diagnosis of candida and under-diagnosis of BV
- Free, confidential home testing for STIs is available online from freetest.me

Microscopy is the most reliable way to make a diagnosis, but it is unlikely to be available in primary care. See algorithm in Figure 10.1.

BOX 10.1 VAGINAL pH TESTING

- Take a swab or cotton bud and rub it along the lateral wall of the vagina, collecting some discharge. Avoid the cervix and the posterior fornix (because of cervical alkaline secretions)
- Rub the swab immediately on to specific narrow-range pH paper (e.g. Simplex Health range 3.8–5.4). Urine dipsticks are not suitable
- The normal vaginal pH in a woman of childbearing age is 4.5 or less (kept acidic by normal lactobacilli)
- pH may be raised because of:
  - Menstrual blood
  - Semen
  - KY jelly
  - BV, Trichomonas vaginalis (TV), gonorrhoea and chlamydia infection
- Candida does not affect the pH
- Individual pH testing kits may be bought OTC

 RED FLAGS

- Suspected severe pelvic inflammatory disease (*admit under Gynaecology*). Look for any of the following:
  - Nausea or vomiting
  - Fever greater than 38°C
  - Systemically unwell/tachycardia
  - Signs of pelvic peritonitis (pain, tenderness and swelling of lower abdomen)
- Systemically unwell plus pregnant, postpartum, after termination of pregnancy or gynaecological procedure (*high risk of sepsis; refer to Gynaecology same-day*)

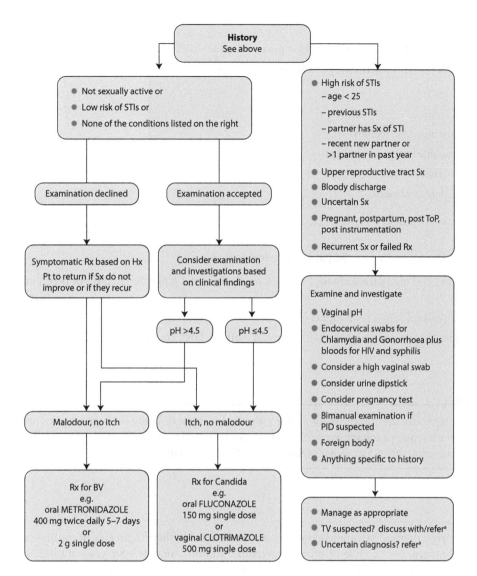

Figure 10.1 Vaginal discharge in women of reproductive years in primary care. Hx: history, PID: pelvic inflammatory disease, Pt: patient, Rx: treatment, Sx: symptoms, ToP: termination of pregnancy. [a]Discuss with or refer to Sexual Health Service. (Adapted from Lazaro, 2013.)

BACTERIAL VAGINOSIS (BV)

Caused by an overgrowth of anaerobic bacteria in the vagina at the expense of the normal commensal lactobacteria. More likely to occur in sexually active women but can occur if sexually inactive. More common in black women, smokers, copper intrauterine device (IUD) users, and those using bubble bath or vaginal douching.

History
- Duration
- Nature of discharge – usually thin and white
- Smell – fishy
- No itching or soreness
- Any previous episodes
- Treatments already tried
- ⚑ Possibility of pregnancy (*associated with late miscarriage, preterm birth, postpartum endometritis*)

Examination (if indicated, see previous section)
- Speculum examination shows thin, smooth, white discharge coating the vagina, no inflammation

Tests

- Offer pH testing (see Box 10.1). The vaginal pH is greater than 4.5 with BV
- Definitive diagnosis requires microscopy at a Sexual Health clinic

Self-care

- Not a sexually transmitted infection
- Avoid douching, bubble bath and antiseptics
- No need to treat sexual partner
- No need to retest after treatment

Prescription

Any one of the following depending on the patient's preference:

- Metronidazole^Q tabs 400 mg twice daily for 7 days. A single dose of 2 g may be used if not pregnant, but relapse rates are higher
- Metronidazole vaginal gel 0.75% for 5 nights (40 g)
- Clindamycin vaginal cream for 7 nights (40 g). Caution – affects latex condoms

RED FLAG

- Pregnant women who are symptomatic with BV should be treated. There is no good evidence to support treating asymptomatic pregnant women, unless they have human immunodeficiency virus (HIV) or other risk factors for pre-term birth (*discuss with Obstetrics or Sexual Health*)

CANDIDA

Up to 20% of women are colonised by candida (a yeast) as a commensal in their vagina (i.e. it causes no symptoms). A change in pH or hormone balance, or a course of broad spectrum antibiotic, may trigger yeast multiplication and symptoms. Approximately 75% of women may have an episode of symptomatic vaginal candidiasis in their lifetime.

History

- Duration
- Colour – usually white, but variable
- Smell – yeasty
- Itch (the characteristic symptom)
- Pain with intercourse
- Any previous episodes
- Timing with menstrual cycle
- Recent broad-spectrum antibiotics
- Diabetes – if so, how well controlled
- Immunosuppressed
- Treatments already tried
- Possibility of pregnancy

Examination (not usually indicated, see previous section)

- Inflamed vulva, maybe fissures
- Speculum examination shows white 'cottage cheese' discharge on cervix and in vagina

Tests

- Offer pH testing (see previous section) to exclude BV. The vaginal pH is normal ($\leq$ 4.5) in a candida infection
- If resistant to treatment, and patient declines Sexual Health referral, take high vaginal swabs (HVS) and ask the laboratory to test for non-albicans candida species
- If recurrent or severe symptoms, arrange fasting plasma glucose or HbA1c (if clinically appropriate) to test for diabetes

Self-care

- Avoid irritating the area with soap, shower gel or bath additives. Use a soap substitute
- Avoid tight-fitting synthetic fabrics
- Buy a clotrimazole pessary or oral fluconazole[PCIQ] capsule (these are equally effective, although clotrimazole may give more rapid relief. The price is similar, although variable; supermarkets usually offer the lowest prices)
- Using clotrimazole cream with the clotrimazole pessary/fluconazole[PCIQ] capsule may relieve external itching more quickly
- Combination packs of clotrimazole cream and pessary (e.g. Canesten Combi®) and clotrimazole cream and fluconazole[PCIQ] capsule (e.g. Canesten Duo®) can be bought over the counter (OTC) more cheaply than through a prescription (as the combination packs entail two prescription charges)
- If itching is severe, consider clotrimazole/hydrocortisone cream instead of clotrimazole cream
- Caution – clotrimazole affects latex condoms
- No need to treat sexual partner, unless they have symptoms
- No evidence to support the use of live yoghourt or probiotics, although they do no harm

---

 BOX 10.2 VAGINAL CANDIDIASIS ("THRUSH") – TREATMENT OPTIONS

First line

C500 = clotrimazole 500 mg pessaries, one at night *or*
F150 = oral fluconazole[PCIQ] 150 mg capsules, one dose

Second line

Try the alternative first-line option (as above).

Third line if both of the previous treatments have failed

C200 = clotrimazole 200 mg pessaries, one at night for 6 nights *or*
F50² = oral fluconazole[PCIQ] 50 mg capsules, two daily for 7 days

---

Prescription

- For uncomplicated infections, follow Box 10.2 above
- If severe or persistent symptoms, give:
  - F150 repeated after 3 days, or
  - C500 repeated after 3 days
- If poorly controlled diabetes or immunosuppression, give:
  - F50², or
  - C200
- If pregnant and symptomatic, give:
  - C200. The patient may prefer to insert the pessary manually
- If recurrent symptoms, reconsider the diagnosis. Offer a prolonged initial treatment course (e.g. F150 repeated after 3 days), then a supply for 'treatment when needed' may be given, or a maintenance treatment plan may be offered for 6 months:
  - Clotrimazole 500 mg pessaries once a week
  - Fluconazole[PCIQ] 150 mg capsules once a week
  - Itraconazole[PCBIQ] 200 mg capsules twice daily for 1 day, once a month

References

Lazaro, N. 2013. *Sexually Transmitted Infections in Primary Care*, 2nd edition. RCGP/BASHH guideline. www.bashhguidelines.org/media/1089/sexually-transmitted-infections-in-primary-care-2013.pdf.

NICE CKS. 2014. Bacterial vaginosis. cks.nice.org.uk/bacterial-vaginosis.

NICE CKS. 2015. Pelvic inflammatory disease. cks.nice.org.uk/pelvic-inflammatory-disease.

NICE CKS. 2016. Candida – female genital. cks.nice.org.uk/candida-female-genital.

Thinkhamrop, J., Hofmeyr, G., Adetoro, O., Lumbiganon, P., and Ota, E. 2015. Antibiotic prophylaxis during the second and third trimester to reduce adverse pregnancy outcomes and morbidity. *Cochrane Database of Systematic Reviews*; (6). Art. No.: CD002250. doi: 10.1002/14651858.CD002250.pub3. *Antibiotic prophylaxis did not reduce the risk of preterm pre-labour rupture of membranes or preterm delivery (apart from in the subgroup of women with a previous preterm birth who had bacterial vaginosis).*

HEAVY MENSTRUAL BLEEDING

This is a common problem; in 50% of women, no underlying cause can be found. Possible diagnoses include fibroids and endometriosis.

History

- Duration and heaviness of this period
- Usual pattern of menstrual cycle
- Clots/flooding
- Dysmenorrhoea
- Contraceptive usage/missed pills
- Was this period late (possible miscarriage?)
- 🚩 Did the period come after 12 months or more of amenorrhoea
- 🚩 Intermenstrual or post-coital bleeding (see section that follows)

Examination

- If bleeding is currently very heavy, check pulse rate and blood pressure (BP) and check for signs of a haematological disorder (e.g. pallor or skin bruises)
- Urgent pelvic examination is not necessary
- Abdominal and pelvic examination is recommended if symptoms suggest underlying pathology, if initial treatment is ineffective, or if a levonorgestrel-releasing intrauterine system (IUS[P]) is being considered

Tests

- Full blood count (FBC) and ferritin should be checked in all women with heavy menstrual bleeding
- Consider checking thyroid status if any symptoms or signs of hypothyroidism such as weight gain, constipation or cold intolerance (fatigue could be driven by anaemia)
- Consider coagulation testing if there is a family history of a clotting disorder, and there has been heavy bleeding since menarche

Self-care

- Explain that there is no link between passing 'clots' in the menstrual blood and internal thrombosis. Patients often worry about this
- Ibuprofen[P] (200–400 mg three times daily for adults) often reduces menstrual flow significantly. It is chemically related to mefenamic acid[PBI] but has a better side effect profile. The more potent NSAID naproxen[PBCI] (500 mg initially, then 250 mg up to three times daily as required for adults) is now available OTC for painful periods
- Tranexamic acid[P] is also usually effective; do not use alongside the combined oral contraceptive because of an increased risk of venous thromboembolism (VTE)
- Iron[I] supplements may be needed if loss has been heavy. The recommended dose to treat iron deficiency is 60 to 120 mg of elemental iron per day for a minimum of three months. Many OTC iron supplements contain much lower doses than this. If gastrointestinal side-effects are a problem, try reducing the dose rather than changing the form of iron

- There are several options for treatment; NICE produce a useful leaflet (see References). The intrauterine system (IUS[P]) is often the best choice

Prescription

- If the above treatment fails, medroxyprogesterone acetate[PC] (10 mg three times daily; *unlicensed indication*) may stop the bleeding within 2 days. A light bleed can occur on discontinuing. Norethisterone[PBC] has traditionally been used for this indication, but although it is a progestogen, it is metabolised to ethinyloestradiol, and the higher doses used for menorrhagia carry an increased risk of VTE comparable to the combined oral contraceptive (COC)

RED FLAGS

- Persistent intermenstrual or post-coital bleeding (*possible STI or carcinoma of cervix; arrange sexual health screen and speculum examination*)
- Palpable abdominal mass (*possible fibroids or carcinoma of uterus or ovary; if not obviously fibroids, 2-week wait cancer referral to Gynaecology*)
- Bleeding after 1 year of amenorrhoea (post-menopausal bleeding) (*possible carcinoma of uterus; refer to Gynaecology urgently if <55 or on 2-week wait if ≥55*)

References

Mansour, D. 2012. Safer prescribing of therapeutic norethisterone for women at risk of venous thromboembolism. *J Fam Plann Reprod Health Care*; 38:148–149. http://jfprhc.bmj.com/content/38/3/148. doi: 10.1136/jfprhc-2012-100345.

NICE CG44. 2016. Heavy menstrual bleeding: Treatment and care for women with heavy periods. www.nice.org.uk/guidance/cg44/ifp/chapter/Treatment-and-care-for-women-with-heavy-periods.

NICE CKS. 2015. Menorrhagia. https://cks.nice.org.uk/menorrhagia.

NICE NG12. 2015. Suspected cancer: Recognition and referral. www.nice.org.uk/guidance/ng12.

INTERMENSTRUAL BLEEDING

History

- Menstrual cycle
- Date of LMP
- Previous episodes
- Sexual history (see beginning of chapter)
- Last smear test and its outcome
- Recent first experience of penetrative sex
- Contraceptive method (if on oral contraceptive, then ask about missed pills/vomiting/enzyme-inducing drugs)
- Hormone replacement therapy (HRT)
- Any possibility of pregnancy
- Fever
- Abdominal pain
- Offensive discharge
- Recent childbirth, termination of pregnancy, gynaecological intervention or miscarriage

Examination

- Not necessary while still bleeding unless red flags present, in which case *refer urgently to Gynaecology or Sexual Health*

Tests

- NAAT test for chlamydia and gonorrhoea
- Consider pregnancy test

Action

- If missed contraceptive pills/vomiting/diarrhoea, see next section
- If recent first experience of penetrative sex, reassure that some bleeding is common

- If missed HRT tablets, resume tablet taking and make appointment if bleeding persists
- Otherwise, make appointment for vaginal examination when bleeding stops

RED FLAGS

- Systemically unwell/fever on background of abdominal pain/offensive discharge (*possible pelvic inflammatory disease; refer same-day to Gynaecology or Sexual Health*)
- Recent childbirth, termination, gynaecological intervention or miscarriage (*possible endometritis; refer urgently to Gynaecology*)
- Pregnant (*may need Obstetrics/Gynaecology referral*)

ORAL CONTRACEPTIVES, DIARRHOEA AND VOMITING

Vomiting and persistent, severe diarrhoea can interfere with the absorption of combined oral contraceptives. If vomiting occurs within 2 hours of taking any oral contraceptive, another pill should be taken as soon as possible. If the replacement pill cannot be kept down, then extra precautions are needed (see Table 10.1).

With COCs, if the illness occurs during the last seven tablets in the pack, the next pill-free interval should be omitted; in the case of everyday (ED) tablets, the inactive ones should be omitted. Consider emergency contraception if sexual intercourse without a condom occurred in the pill-free interval or in the first week of pill taking.

In cases of vomiting or persistent severe diarrhoea, additional precautions should be used during illness and also after recovery (see Table 10.1).

Table 10.1 Need for extra precautions with different types of oral contraceptives

Classification	Type	Diarrhoea/vomiting persisting longer than …	Continue extra precautions after recovery for …
COC	Qlaira	12 hours	9 days[a]
	Others	24 hours	7 days
POP	Desogestrel	12 hours	2 days
	Others	3 hours	2 days

[a] No extra precautions are needed for unabsorbed inactive white tablets of Qlaira.

ANTIBIOTICS AND ORAL CONTRACEPTIVES

The Faculty of Sexual and Reproductive Healthcare (FSRH) issued guidance in 2011 to bring UK clinical practice in line with WHO guidance issued the previous year. In a review of the evidence for an interaction between antibiotics and contraceptives, the FSRH concluded that: 'Overall, the evidence does not support reduced combined oral contraception efficacy with non-enzyme-inducing antibiotics. Additional contraceptive precautions are not required during or after courses of antibiotics that do not induce enzymes'. The same advice applies to progestogen-only methods.

This has remained unchanged in FSRH guidance since 2011. The antibiotics that we recommend for the treatment of minor illness do not induce liver enzymes, so extra contraceptive precautions are not necessary.

Reference

Faculty of Sexual & Reproductive Healthcare and RCOG. 2017. Drug interactions with hormonal contraception. www.fsrh.org/documents/ceu-clinical-guidance-drug-interactions-with-hormonal/.

EMERGENCY CONTRACEPTION (EC)

History

- If under 16, check if Fraser competent, her ability to consent to sex and age of her partner (see Box 10.3)
- Date of LMP
- Time since unprotected sexual intercourse (UPSI)
- Sexual history (see beginning of chapter)

- Risk of sexually transmitted infection (by definition, if EC is needed, the woman is at risk of an STI)
- Previous UPSI this cycle may render oral treatment ineffective – consider copper intrauterine contraceptive device[P] (IUCD[P])
- Previous emergency contraception this cycle
- Usual contraceptive method and any problems e.g. missed pills, late injection
- On enzyme-inducing medication, for example, carbamazepine, phenytoin, rifampicin, or herbal preparations such as St John's wort
- Breastfeeding
- Past history of porphyria or asthma (this is relevant to prescribing)
- Ongoing need for contraception
- 🚩 Risk of having had non-consensual sexual intercourse

BOX 10.3 LEGAL ISSUES AROUND PROVIDING EMERGENCY CONTRACEPTION TO THOSE UNDER 16

In the United Kingdom, the legal age of consent to sexual activity is 16. One in three young people have had sexual intercourse before the age of 16, but sexual activity under the age of consent is an offence, even if consensual. Offences are considered more serious (statutory rape) when the person is younger than 13 years. In England and Wales, it is legal to provide contraceptive advice and treatment to young people without parental consent, provided that the practitioner is satisfied that the Fraser criteria for competence are met:

- The young person understands the practitioner's advice
- The young person cannot be persuaded to inform their parents or will not allow the practitioner to inform the parents that contraceptive advice has been sought
- The young person is likely to begin or to continue having intercourse with or without contraceptive treatment
- Unless she receives contraceptive advice or treatment, the young person's physical or mental health (or both) are likely to suffer
- The young person's best interest requires the practitioner to give contraceptive advice or treatment (or both) without parental consent

All available methods of emergency contraception should be offered, regardless of age, as the risk of an unwanted pregnancy outweighs that of the contraceptive.

Note: Child protection issues should be taken into account – it is important to be assured that sex has been consensual and is not occurring in an incestuous relationship. If it is suspected that force has been used or that sexual abuse has occurred, you have a duty to follow national and local safeguarding procedures.

Reference

Faculty of Sexual and Reproductive Healthcare (FSRH). 2010. FSRH clinical guidance: Contraceptive choices for young people. www.fsrh.org/standards-and-guidance/documents/cec-ceu-guidance-young-people-mar-2010/.

Self-care

Indication for EC

- Emergency contraception is advised following intercourse when:
  - No contraception has been used *or*
  - A barrier contraceptive failed *or*
  - The COC is used but would be less effective because two or more pills were missed (more than 48 hours late in week 1) *or*
  - The POP is used but would be less effective because >27 hours since the last pill (>36 hours late for desogestrel-only pill) *or*
  - The injectable progestogen is likely to be less effective as the last injection of medroxyprogesterone acetate was ≥14 weeks ago

  and, if there has been a recent pregnancy:
  - It has been 21 days or more since childbirth *or*
  - It has been 5 days or more since termination of pregnancy or miscarriage
- Different EC methods have different rates of success in preventing pregnancy (Table 10.2)

- An emergency copper IUCD is the most reliable option for EC, about 20 times more effective than the oral methods. It provides ongoing contraception and can be fitted up to day 19 of a 28-day cycle
- Emergency oral contraception is provided free of charge by sexual health clinics and General Practitioner (GP) practices, also by all pharmacies in Scotland and Wales and some pharmacies in England and Northern Ireland
- Women aged 16 or over can buy levonorgestrel[P] and ulipristal[PB] OTC from most UK pharmacies
- Oral EC may cause nausea. Seek help if vomiting within 2 hours of taking levonorgestrel or 3 hours of taking ulipristal[PB] (see Cautions below)

Table 10.2 Effectiveness of different EC methods in 1,000 women at risk

	No EC	Levonorgestrel	Ulipristal	Copper IUCD
Pregnancies	80	26	18	1

Advice
- After taking EC, many women ovulate later in the cycle. They must be advised of the need for ongoing contraception
- Use condoms, or do not have penetrative sex, until next period, which may be early or late
- Pregnancy test is recommended if next period more than 1 week late
- No known adverse effect on foetus if pregnancy occurs, but ectopic pregnancy is possible. Seek advice if lower abdominal pain (different from usual period pain) or period is lighter than usual
- Consider long-term contraception, STI screening and safe sex advice

Prescription if IUCD fit declined:
- The FSRH guideline states that EC providers should advise women that ulipristal[PB] has been demonstrated to be more effective than levonorgestrel (see Table 10.2). However, it is also more expensive. Some Clinical Commissioning Groups (CCGs) restrict its use, although it has been argued that it is more cost effective overall due to greater efficacy. We recommend prescribing ulipristal to all, but if your prescribing is restricted then we suggest the following:
  - If UPSI occurred within previous 72 hours, a woman weighs <70 kg, and is not in her most fertile phase (the 5 days before ovulation, that is, days 9–14 of a 28-day cycle), prescribe one levonorgestrel[P] 1.5 mg tablet. If breastfeeding, she should take the dose immediately after breastfeeding and allow 8 hours before recommencing
  - If UPSI occurred between 72 and 120 hours previously, weight ≥70 kg, or in her fertile phase, prescribe one ulipristal[PB] 30 mg tablet. If breastfeeding, she should discard the milk for 7 days
- For those on enzyme-inducing medicines, a copper IUCD[P] is the best option, but if the woman still declines, prescribe two tablets of levonorgestrel[P] 1.5 mg, to be taken together. A double dose of ulipristal[PB] is not recommended
- Advise that the EC dose should be taken as soon as possible, as the earlier it is taken, the more effective it is
- Also offer 'quick-start' of a long-term method of contraception, but remember that the effect of ulipristal[PB] may be reduced if the woman takes progestogen in the next 5 days

Cautions
- Oral EC is unlikely to be effective if taken after ovulation. See FSRH (2017) for more information and a useful algorithm
- If a patient vomits within 2 hours of taking levonorgestrel[P] or within 3 hours of taking ulipristal[PB], give a replacement prescription, plus domperidone[PIQ] 10 mg to be taken 30 minutes before EC dose
- For complex problems, contact the National Sexual Health Helpline at 0300 123 7123 (Mon–Fri, 9 a.m.–8 p.m.)

References

Bayer, L.L., Edelman, A.B., Caughey, A.B., and Rodriguez, M.I. 2013. The price of emergency contraception in the United States: What is the cost effectiveness of ulipristal acetate versus single-dose levonorgestrel? *Contraception*; 87(3):385–390. www.contraceptionjournal.org/article/S0010-7824(12)00800-1/fulltext. doi: 10.1016/j.contraception.2012.08.034.

FSRH. 2017. CEU clinical guidance: Emergency contraception. www.fsrh.org/documents/ceu-clinical-guidance-emergency-contraception-march-2017/.

Glasier, A.F., Cameron, S.T., Fine, P.M., Logan, S.J.S., Casale, W., Van Horn, J., Sogor, L. et al. 2010. Ulipristal acetate versus levonorgestrel for emergency contraception: A randomised non-inferiority trial and meta-analysis. *Lancet*; 375(9714):555–562. doi: 10.1016/S0140-6736(10)60101-8.

DELAYING A PERIOD

A woman whose period is due when she is on holiday, or taking part in a religious or sporting event, may request medication to delay her period. The traditional and licensed treatment is norethisterone[PBC] 5 mg three times daily, started 3 days before the period is expected to begin. A light period should occur 2–3 days after stopping the course.

Although norethisterone is a progestogen, it is metabolised to ethinyloestradiol, and the higher doses used to delay a period carry an increased risk of VTE comparable to the COC. Women who request medication to delay a period should therefore be assessed in the same way as those wishing to start the COC, and if at increased risk of VTE, they should be prescribed medroxyprogesterone acetate[PC] 10 mg three times daily instead (*unlicensed indication*). Neither of these medicines are contraceptive at these doses. Flights of more than 4 hours double the risk of VTE, but the absolute risk is low: one event per 6,000 flights.

If a woman is already taking the COC, then she may delay her withdrawal bleed by omitting the pill-free interval and moving straight onto the next pill packet, but if she is taking a type that contains placebo tablets (e.g. an ED formulation), then she will need preparation-specific advice.

References

Izadi, M., Alemzadeh-Ansari, M.J., Kazemisaleh, D., and Jonidi, N. 2014. Venous thromboembolism following travel. *Int J Travel Med Glob Health*; 2(1):23–30. www.ijtmgh.com/article_33271_686fb55f40959626391cd33b0901c577.pdf.

Mansour, D. 2012. Safer prescribing of therapeutic norethisterone for women at risk of venous thromboembolism. *J Fam Plann Reprod Health Care*; 38:148–149. http://jfprhc.bmj.com/content/38/3/148. doi: 10.1136/jfprhc-2012-100345.

NICE CKS. 2013. DVT prevention for travellers. cks.nice.org.uk/dvt-prevention-for-travellers.

MASTITIS

In lactating women, blocked milk flow is the main cause of mastitis. Milk leaks into the surrounding tissues, where cytokines cause inflammation. If milk products pass into the bloodstream, they can produce malaise and fever, even if there is no infection. Without effective milk drainage, staphylococcal infection is likely to develop, which may lead to abscess formation.

In non-lactating women, smokers are at highest risk, and the responsible bacteria are different. There is no good research to guide the prescription of antibiotics in this situation.

History
- Lactating
- Smoking history
- Fever
- Location of pain and character
- Redness of breast
- Is this recurrent?
- Was onset while in hospital?
- Nipple discharge
- 🚩 Immunosuppressed

Examination
- Temperature
- Pulse rate
- Record area of redness – often wedge-shaped
- Examine nipples for inflammation or visible discharge
- 🚩 Check for any suggestion of an abscess (red, fluctuant lump)

Self-care
- If lactating:
  - See a breastfeeding advisor
  - Continue to breastfeed from both sides, offering the affected side first

- Express any remaining milk
- Paracetamol or ibuprofen[P] to relieve pain
- Treat any nipple problem (e.g. candida)
- Warm compress, warm bath or shower
- Rest (as much as a newborn/infant allows)
- Do not wear a bra at night
- Seek further advice if worsening or not improving after 48 hours

Tests

- Breast milk culture if severe or recurrent, hospital-acquired infection or deep burning pain

Action (See box 10.4)

 BOX 10.4   ANTIBIOTICS FOR MASTITIS

Prescribe an antibiotic if:

- Severe symptoms
- Immunosuppressed (including diabetes)
- Yellow discharge from nipple
- Not improving after 12–24 hours despite effective milk removal (consider a delayed prescription)

Antibiotic choice

- If lactating:
  - Flucloxacillin 500 mg four times daily for 10–14 days
  - Clarithromycin[PIQ] 500 mg twice daily for 10–14 days if allergic to penicillin
- If not lactating:
  - Co-amoxiclav 500/125 mg three times daily for 10–14 days
  - Clarithromycin[PIQ] 500 mg twice daily plus metronidazole[Q] 500 mg three times daily for 10–14 days if allergic to penicillin

 RED FLAGS

- Signs of sepsis or immunosuppressed (*admit under Surgical*)
- Abscess suspected (*ultrasound and aspiration may be needed; admit under Surgical*)
- Underlying mass (*possible breast cancer; refer on 2-week wait to Breast Clinic*)

References

Dixon, J.M., and Khan, L.R. 2011. Treatment of breast infection. *BMJ*; 342:d396. doi: 10.1136/bmj.d396.
NICE CKS. 2015. Mastitis and breast abscess. cks.nice.org.uk/mastitis-and-breast-abscess.

NIPPLE PAIN

Pain during breastfeeding is usually due to problems with attachment of the baby to the breast.

History

- One or both sides affected
- Severity, type and timing of pain
- Use of nipple shield
- Does baby have tongue tie, oral thrush or nappy rash?

- Does nipple blanch during feeds or when it is cold? If so, does it become red afterwards?
- Discharge from nipple

Examination

- Inverted nipples
- Loss of colour in the nipples or areola
- Pink or red colour, flaking, shininess, crusting
- Fissure

Possible causes

- Sore and fissured nipples may be due to friction and poor positioning (most common)
  - Problems usually start early; pain occurs during feed and may be severe
  - Self-care: see breastfeeding advisor. Apply Vaseline© to any broken skin
- Candida
  - Usually bilateral
  - Delayed by a few weeks after childbirth, unless woman has had recent candida infection
  - Burning and itching
  - Nipples appear pale, fissured or normal
  - Self-care: apply miconazole[I] 2% cream to nipples after each feed for 2 weeks; wipe away any remaining cream before next feed
  - Treat baby with miconazole[I] oral gel (see section on Oral Candidiasis in Chapter 5)
- Bacterial infection
  - Yellow discharge from nipple
  - Persistent fissure
  - Prescription: sodium fusidate ointment after each feed for 7 days. If severe, give oral flucloxacillin (or clarithromycin[PIQ] if patient is allergic to penicillin)
- Eczema
  - Burning and itching
  - Redness, vesicles, crusting or scaling
  - Base of nipple may be unaffected
  - Self-care: consider allergy to creams or new food given to baby. Avoid soap, shower gel, and so forth. Apply hydrocortisone or Eumovate® ointment twice daily after feeds until recovered; wipe away any remaining cream before next feed
- Raynaud's disease of nipple
  - Nipple may blanch during feed or when cold, then become red
  - Intermittent pain persists after feeding, when cold and may be severe
  - Self-care: keep warm. Avoid smoking and caffeine
  - Prescription: nifedipine[PC] capsules 5 mg three times a day for 2 weeks (*unlicensed indication*). May be continued if necessary

RED FLAG

- Unilateral eczema not responding to treatment (*possible breast cancer; 2-week wait referral to Breast Clinic*)

Reference

NICE CKS. 2017. Breastfeeding problems. cks.nice.org.uk/breastfeeding-problems.

CHAPTER 11

Mental health

People who present with minor illness may also have underlying mental health problems. Sometimes they may present these openly to you, but more often they will tell you about their physical symptoms because they often perceive these as being more acceptable. You do not need to be an expert in mental health to pick up these problems, and it is not necessary to make a definite diagnosis in order to help; often in primary care the problems arise from relationships, work, housing issues or debt, for which you may be able to suggest appropriate local or national services. Whatever the problems, the patient's ability to cope can be improved by encouraging them to exercise (outdoors if possible) and to learn techniques that enable them to deeply relax.

DEPRESSION

This is a very common condition in which physical symptoms are often presented initially. Be aware that it may be an underlying problem in any consultation. Any age group can be affected. The diagnosis is easily overlooked in older people, although it is often the underlying issue for memory disturbance. Depression in children requires specialist management.

There is debate about the possibility that depression could be an adaptive behaviour in response to life circumstances. This has created a new specialty called evolutionary psychology (see http://journals.sagepub.com/home/evp). Although not established, such an approach may be more helpful to the patient than assuming depression is a disease that afflicts people when there is no clear pathophysiology.

History

Active, empathetic listening is of utmost importance. You may be the first to hear the patient's story.

- How long the patient has felt low
- Any specific reason or trigger identified, for example, bereavement, childbirth, relationship difficulties, financial worries, stress at work
- Core symptoms: feelings of sadness, lack of interest/enjoyment in life. Ask 'what are you looking forward to?'
- Appetite (may be overeating or undereating) or weight changes
- Sleep disturbance/fatigue. Early morning waking is typically described
- Feelings of worthlessness or guilt
- Loss of concentration/poor memory
- Ask: 'How will you know when you are better? What will you be doing that you aren't doing now?'
- Previous episodes and treatment, and what helped them to resolve their problems
- Medication, alcohol intake, recreational drugs
- Risk factors, for example, previous history, chronic illness, dementia
- Adequacy of social support, living conditions
- Safeguarding issues
- NICE recommends two initial questions to consider when depression is suspected, but be aware that these can be leading questions, which reduces their diagnostic power:
  - During the last month, have you often been bothered by feeling down, depressed or hopeless?
  - During the last month, have you often been bothered by having little interest or pleasure in doing things?
- ⚑ Thoughts of death: 'Have you ever felt that life wasn't worth living?' (passive suicidal ideation). If any such thoughts, ask 'have you ever felt like ending your own life' (active suicidal ideation), and if so, what has stopped them thus far from acting upon this (protective factors). Having a plan for how they would end their life suggests that they are at even higher risk. The burden of mental illness affects women and men, but 75% of the suicides in the United Kingdom in 2015 were men. Risk factors include substance misuse, recent stressful life event (bereavement, loss of job, divorce) and exposure to another person's suicide/personal or family history of suicide attempts

Examination

- Note patient's appearance – any signs of self-neglect?
- Observe body language, especially moist eyes, trembling lower lip, avoiding eye contact

Test

- Ask patient to complete a validated questionnaire: Patient Health Questionnaire 9 (https://patient.info/doctor/patient-health-questionnaire-phq-9) or Hospital Anxiety and Depression Scale which, despite its name, has been validated for use in primary care

Self-care

- Invite patient to consider practical problem-solving, for example, change of job – but avoid being directive
- Daily exercise, especially walking outdoors with a relative, friend or dog, can help
- Try to resume activities previously enjoyed. The cycle of poor motivation leading to abandoning previously enjoyable activities, which then further compounds low mood and poor motivation, is particularly destructive
- Consider learning relaxation techniques (depression is often driven by anxiety)
- If alcohol and substance misuse are part of the problem, offer a referral to the appropriate specialist service
- Ensure a regular intake of healthy food, including oily fish and whole grains
- Avoid excessive caffeine
- Self-help books and websites (see 'resources for patients' that follows)
- Moodgym® (www.moodgym.com.au) is an online self-help program designed to help people with depression and anxiety. It teaches skills based on cognitive behavioural therapy (CBT)
- Most areas allow self-referral to local psychological therapy services and offer a range of interventions including counselling and CBT

Action

- Empathise and be positive about recovery
- If applicable, remind the patient that they have already learnt coping strategies that have previously helped them
- Recommend restorative sleep techniques (see next section on Insomnia)
- If taking regular medication, check side effects in British National Formulary (BNF). Benzodiazepines, steroids, simvastatin, opioids such as codeine, varenicline (Champix® for smoking cessation), propranolol, anticonvulsants and hormonal medications including contraceptives are some of the drugs that may precipitate depression
- If work-related stress, would time off, limited duties or reduced hours help?
- If mild-moderate symptoms, offer referral/self-referral to local psychological therapy services for low intensity psychological interventions (e.g. guided self-help, group-based peer support, computerised CBT). If symptoms are mild but persistent then offer the same
- If moderate or severe symptoms, offer referral for high-intensity interventions (e.g. group or individual CBT) and consider referral to a General Practitioner (GP) for antidepressants – emphasise that these are not addictive. There is usually a 3-week delay before positive effects are seen, and the course can last several months
- All patients should be followed up within 2 weeks
- St John's wort was not recommended by NICE because of lack of standardisation of products and drug interactions. However, there is a considerable body of evidence to show that it is as effective as selective serotonin reuptake inhibitors (SSRIs), and it avoids the perceived stigma of an antidepressant prescription. It interacts with many drugs, notably combined oral contraceptives, warfarin, amlodipine, triptans (for migraine) and anticonvulsants. See Interactions section of BNF

RED FLAGS

- If suicidal thoughts are expressed, an urgent risk assessment should be made by an experienced practitioner as to whether an immediate referral to a crisis team or A&E should be offered
- Active suicidal ideation (thoughts about harming oneself) is considered a higher risk than passive suicidal ideation (thoughts of life not being worth living), particularly if associated with plans for how it would be done
- If patient declines referral, give contact details of the Samaritans (currently 116123, www.samaritans.org) and discuss with a senior colleague afterwards

References

Apaydin, E., Maher, A., Shanman, R., Booth, M., Miles, J., Sorbero, M., and Hempel, S. 2016. A systematic review of St. John's wort for major depressive disorder. *Systematic Reviews*; 5:148. doi: 10.1186/s13643-016-0325-2. *SJW monotherapy for mild and moderate depression is superior to placebo in improving depression symptoms and not significantly different from antidepressant medication. However, evidence of heterogeneity and a lack of research on severe depression reduce the quality of the evidence.*

Köhler, O., Benros, M.E., Nordentoft, M., Farkouh, M.E., Iyengar, R.L., Mors, O., and Krogh, J. 2014. Effect of anti-inflammatory treatment on depression, depressive symptoms, and adverse effects: A systematic review and meta-analysis of randomized clinical trials. *JAMA Psychiatry*; 71(12):1381–1391. http://jamanetwork.com/journals/jamapsychiatry/fullarticle/1916904. doi: 10.1001/jamapsychiatry.2014.1611. *There is currently much interest in the role of anti-inflammatory medicines such as celecoxib in treating depression.*

NICE CG90. 2009. The treatment and management of depression in adults. www.nice.org.uk/guidance/CG90.

Wani, A.L., Bhat, S.A., and Ara, A. 2015. Omega-3 fatty acids and the treatment of depression: A review of scientific evidence. *Integr Med Res*; 4(3):132–141. www.sciencedirect.com/science/article/pii/S2213422015005387. doi: 10.1016/j.imr.2015.07.003. *This article suggests that omega-3 supplements may be helpful for depressed people whose diet is poor.*

INSOMNIA

Insomnia is common and subjective. Some people only require 4 or 5 hours of sleep a night, whereas others need 10 hours or more. The amount of sleep required tends to lessen with age and with lower activity levels. A 'good night's sleep' is not the same for everyone. Almost everyone can have periods of insomnia at some stage. Tiredness is often considered the enemy, but building up a healthy level of tiredness over the course of a day can promote better sleep at night.

History

- What is the patient's concern about the sleep pattern?
- When did the problem start, and what was happening to them at that time?
- What is the sleep pattern?
  - Difficulty getting off to sleep
  - Recurrent waking during the night
  - Early morning waking, feeling unrefreshed
- Does the patient take daytime naps?
- Reported to snore with gasping or restlessness during the night (particularly if overweight)
- Is the bedroom comfortable, quiet and dark?
- What is done to try to 'wind down' before sleep? (do they watch television, browse the Internet, send text messages, read a book?)
- Any symptoms of depression (see previous section)
- General health
- Medication
- Caffeine, nicotine, alcohol, recreational drugs
- Occupation – for example, shift work, stressful
- What are the patient's expectations – explore their ideas. What do they feel keeps them awake? Why are they coming to see you now? What do they think you can do about it?

Consider causes

- Physical: pain, itching, shortness of breath, nocturia, indigestion/gastro-oesophageal reflux, tinnitus, discomfort
- Physiological: shift work, jet lag, pregnancy, irregular meals, low light levels during the time awake, bright artificial light in the evening (blue light is particularly implicated in circadian regulation; hence the 'night modes' now seen on electronic devices to reduce blue light exposure in the evening)
- Psychological: emotional upsets, worries, bereavement
- Psychiatric: especially depression, hypomania
- Pathological: sleep apnoea, restless legs syndrome, heart failure

- Pharmacological: is patient on any medication possibly causing insomnia, for example, SSRIs, bupropion, lamotrigine, propranolol, corticosteroids, salbutamol, theophylline, pseudoephedrine or laxatives, or taking excessive caffeinated drinks, alcohol, recreational drugs or nicotine
- Social: new baby, enuretic child, partner who has nocturia or who snores

Examination

- Look for agitation, depressed affect, 'washed out' appearance
- Note if body mass index (BMI) >30 (associated with sleep apnoea syndrome)

Self-care

- Consider keeping a sleep diary, which can be downloaded free from http://sleepeducation.org/docs/default-document-library/sleep-diary.pdf
- Try to keep to regular times for going to bed and waking up
- There is only a certain amount of sleep an individual needs in 24 hours. If wanting to sleep more at night, avoid napping during the day
- Don't lie in after a poor night's sleep. Allow the tiredness to be used as 'fuel' for the next night's sleep and to help establish a routine
- Avoid caffeine, nicotine and alcohol within 6 hours of going to bed
- Consider giving up caffeine altogether
- Regular exercise is helpful but not within 4 hours of bedtime
- Try not to eat a heavy meal late at night
- A bedtime ritual (e.g. warm bath, milky drink) may help
- Try to relax before going to bed. Relaxation exercises or training (e.g. hypnotherapy) can be helpful; also yoga, tai chi, meditation, reading and listening to relaxing music
- Keep the bedroom quiet, dark and at a comfortable temperature (usually cooler than other rooms)
- Only use the bedroom for sleep and sex. Banish the television
- Don't keep checking the time throughout the night. Reading a book and watching the page numbers steadily rise can be just as frustrating and is best avoided
- Don't lie in bed awake for more than roughly 20 minutes – it is better to get up and do something productive and then go back to bed when you feel sleepy
- Don't drive if you feel sleepy
- Over-the-counter remedies (such as Nytol®) may contain sedative antihistamines that are temporarily effective but often cause morning drowsiness, or a herb such as valerian, which has not been shown to be effective. They are not recommended
- The website www.sleepeducation.org has useful self-care advice
- A digital CBT program called Sleepio® (www.sleepio.com) has some evidence for improving insomnia. It is available for a subscription fee

Action

- If resulting from work-related stress, would time off, limited duties or reduced hours help?
- Consider adjusting the timing of medications if these are suspected to be affecting sleep

Prescription

- Hypnotic drugs such as zopiclone[PBCI] or temazepam[PBCI] may cause addiction, daytime drowsiness, unsteadiness (with a risk of falls for frail or elderly people) and rebound insomnia on stopping. They are best avoided if possible
- If essential, give zopiclone[PBCI] 3.75 mg tablets or temazepam[PBCI] 10 mg tablets, one on alternate nights for a maximum of 14 days. Warn that they may impair driving the next morning and that alcohol should be avoided when they are used. Make it clear that this is a one-off prescription
- Zopiclone[PBCI] has a superior effect on sleep architecture to temazepam[PBCI], but it is more likely to cause driving impairment the next morning in the elderly (based on 7.5 mg zopiclone vs 20 mg temazepam) (Leufkens et al., 2009; Rudisill et al., 2016)

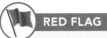

RED FLAG

- Obese and reporting snoring and excessive tiredness (*may need assessment for sleep apnoea; refer to senior colleague*)

References

Espie, C.A., Kyle, S.D., Williams, C., Ong, J.C., Douglas, N.J., Hames, P., and Brown, J.S. 2012. A randomized, placebo-controlled trial of online cognitive behavioral therapy for chronic insomnia disorder delivered via an automated media-rich web application. *Sleep*; 35(6):769–781.

Fernandez-San-Martin, M., Masa-Font, R., Palacios-Soler, L., Sancho-Gomez, P., Calbo-Caldentey, C., and Flores-Mateo, G. 2010. Effectiveness of valerian on insomnia: A meta-analysis of randomized placebo-controlled trials. *Sleep Medicine*; 11(6):505–511. www. crd.york.ac.uk/crdweb/ShowRecord.asp?LinkFrom=OAI&ID=12010004709. *The results suggest that valerian may cause a subjective improvement for insomnia, although its effectiveness was not demonstrated with quantitative or objective measurements.*

Hemmeter, U., Müller, M., Bischof, R., Annen, B., and Holsboer-Trachsler, E. 2000. Effect of zopiclone and temazepam on sleep EEG parameters, psychomotor and memory functions in healthy elderly volunteers. *Psychopharmacology*; 147(4):384–396. https://link. springer.com/article/10.1007%2Fs002130050007?LI=true.

Leufkens, T.R., and Vermeeren, A. 2009. Highway driving in the elderly the morning after bedtime use of hypnotics: A comparison between temazepam 20 mg, zopiclone 7.5 mg, and placebo. *J Clin Pharmacol*; 29(5):432–438.

NICE CKS. 2015. Insomnia. cks.nice.org.uk/insomnia#!scenario.

Mets, M.A., Volkerts, E.R., Olivier, B., and Verster, J.C. 2010. Effect of hypnotic drugs on body balance and standing steadiness. *Sleep Med Rev*; 14(4):259–267. www.smrv-journal.com/article/S1087-0792(09)00118-X/fulltext. doi: 10.1016/j.smrv.2009.10.008.

Rudisill, T.M., Zhu, M., Kelley, G.A., Pilkerton, C., and Rudisill, B.R. 2016. Medication use and the risk of motor vehicle collisions among licensed drivers: A systematic review. *Accident Analysis & Prevention*; 96:255–270.

West, K.E., Jablonski, M.R., Warfield, B., Cecil, K.S., James, M., Ayers, M.A., Maida, J. et al. 2011. Blue light from light-emitting diodes elicits a dose-dependent suppression of melatonin in humans. *J Appl Physiol*; 110(3):619–626.

ANXIETY/PANIC ATTACKS/PHOBIAS

History

Remember to use active, empathetic listening. Disclosing anxiety and phobias (which are often irrational in nature) can be much more difficult for patients than talking about physical symptoms – be careful not to appear to pass any judgment or to trivialise the problem.

- Why have they come? Why today?
- Recent problems: at work, at home, with family or partner, financial
- Symptoms: feeling on edge or restless, dizziness, tiredness, palpitations, dry mouth, excessive sweating, weight loss, urinary frequency, sleep disturbance
- Panic attacks
- Previous mental health problems and how they resolved them
- Caffeine, alcohol, recreational drugs
- Medication: decongestants, salbutamol, corticosteroids

Examination

- Observe body language, especially tremor
- Consider checking pulse rate if organic causes are suspected

Tests

- Consider taking blood for thyroid function tests, if not recently done

Self-care

- Think about practical problem-solving, for example, a change of job
- Daily exercise, especially walking outdoors with a relative, friend or dog, can help

- Reduce or stop intake of caffeine, alcohol and recreational drugs
- Relaxation exercises or training (e.g. hypnotherapy) can be helpful; also yoga, tai chi, meditation, reading and listening to relaxing music
- Recommend self-help books and websites (see section at the end of this chapter)
- Moodgym® (www.moodgym.com.au) is an online self-help program designed to help people with depression and anxiety. It teaches skills based on cognitive behaviour therapy

Action
- Recommend restorative sleep techniques (see earlier section on Insomnia)
- If work-related stress, would time off, limited duties or reduced hours help?
- Empathise and be positive about recovery
- If panic attacks, strongly reassure that they will not cause physical harm such as a heart attack
- Remind patient of any previously learnt coping strategies that have helped them
- Explain the limitations of drug treatment for anxiety
- Explain local arrangements for accessing mental health interventions. Most areas allow people to self-refer to psychological therapy services

Reference
NICE CG113. 2011. Generalised anxiety disorder in adults: Management in primary, secondary and community care. www.nice.org.uk/guidance/cg113.

HYPERVENTILATION

Over-breathing lowers the blood carbon dioxide level. This in turn reduces the transfer of oxygen to the brain, which may cause dizziness and headache, and disturbs blood chemistry ('respiratory alkalosis').

History
- Episodes of being 'unable to take a deep enough breath'
- Absence of other respiratory symptoms, for example, cough/malaise
- Precipitating stress
- Previous episodes
- Chest discomfort
- Tingling around mouth, hands and feet
- In severe cases, spasm of hands and feet (tetany)
- Agoraphobia and panic disorder (50% hyperventilate)
- Asthma (up to 30% hyperventilate)

Examination (to exclude respiratory disease)
- Observe respiration – often irregular or sighing, using upper chest muscles
- Note the ratio of inspiration time to expiration time:
  - Normally about 1:2
  - In asthma, expiration may be prolonged and through pursed lips
  - In hyperventilation, inspiration may be more energetic, and expiration is not prolonged
- Examine chest:
  - Check percussion and that breath sounds are equal on both sides (to exclude pneumothorax)
  - Check for wheeze (this would suggest asthma)
- Record peak flow – should be normal (if low, see section on Asthma in Chapter 4)

Test

- Pulse oximetry to demonstrate oxygen level ≥95% (in hyperventilation, the level may be higher than normal for the person, at 99–100%)

Action

- Explain the problem. Reassure that tingling in arms and hands is not a symptom of a heart attack
- If acute, ask patient to breathe slowly in and out of paper bag, or put hands on head to splint upper chest
- Show patient how to breathe using the diaphragm
- Suggest yoga (breathing exercises and relaxation are both likely to be helpful)
- Relaxation exercises/hypnotherapy may lower the underlying emotional arousal

References

Ito, H., Yokoyama, I., Iida, H., Kinoshita, T., Hatazawa, J., and Shimosegawa, E. 2000. Regional differences in cerebral vascular response to P_aco_2 changes in humans measured by positron emission tomography. *Journal of Cerebral Blood Flow & Metabolism*; 20:1264–1270. http://journals.sagepub.com/doi/abs/10.1097/00004647-200008000-00011. doi: 10.1097/00004647-200008000-00011. *Evidence that low carbon dioxide levels reduce oxygen uptake by the brain.*

Patient.info. 2017. Hyperventilation. https://patient.info/doctor/hyperventilation.

SELF-CARE RESOURCES FOR MENTAL HEALTH

Books

Your local library may have a 'Books on Prescription' scheme with recommended titles and online resources.

- Bradley, D., and Thomas, M. 2011. *Hyperventilation Syndrome: Breathing Pattern Disorders and How to Overcome Them.* Kyle Books. ISBN-13: 978-0857830296
- Griffin, J., and Tyrell, I. 2004. *How to Lift Depression Fast.* HG Publishing. ISBN-13: 978-1899398416
- Griffin, J., and Tyrell, I. 2006. *How to Master Anxiety: All You Need to Know to Overcome Stress, Panic Attacks, Trauma, Phobias, Obsessions and More.* HG Publishing. ISBN-13 978-1899398812
- Johnstone, M. 2007. *I Had a Black Dog.* Robinson Publishing. ISBN-13: 978-184529589. *A cartoon book – a picture is worth a thousand words*
- Skynner, R., and Cleese, J. 1993. *Families and How to Survive Them.* Cedar Books. ISBN-13: 978-0749314101. *For those struggling with family dynamics*

Apps

Phone apps for mindfulness and breathing techniques may be helpful, for example, Headspace and Breath2Relax. They do not require a large time commitment and are free or low cost.

Websites

- Living Life to the Full: www.llttf.com. *Free online CBT and other useful resources*
- Human Givens Institute: www.hgi.org.uk. *Explanation of how unmet emotional needs can cause many mental health problems*
- Royal College of Psychiatrists: www.rcpsych.ac.uk/healthadvice. *Information leaflets in a range of languages*
- Moodgym: moodgym.com.au. *Online self-help (based on CBT) for depression and anxiety*

Agencies

- Relate, for relationship difficulties, www.relate.org.uk, 0300 100 1234
- Drinkaware, www.drinkaware.co.uk
- Drinkline–National Alcohol Helpline, 0300 123 1110
- Citizens' Advice (particularly helpful for debt or benefit problems)
- National Debtline offers free, confidential and independent help over the phone or via webchat for people in England, Scotland and Wales. You can also download sample letters from their website: 0808 808 4000, www.nationaldebtline.co.uk

- Civil Legal Advice (CLA). If you qualify for legal aid and live in England or Wales, CLA can provide free help or legal advice over the phone about debt, housing, employment, education, welfare benefits and tax credits. 0845 345 4 345, www.gov.uk/civil-legal-advice
- Samaritans, a listening ear for all types of problems. Phone 116123 or see www.samaritans.org
- Cruse, for bereavement. 0844 477 9400, www.cruse.org.uk
- Domestic Violence Helpline. Freephone 0808 2000 247(24 hours), www.womensaid.org.uk
- Campaign Against Living Miserably (CALM), charity dedicated to preventing male suicide, 0800 58 58 58 www.thecalmzone.net
- Health Visitor (for parents of children – age range seen varies by region, will always include under 5 years, but may extend up to 19 years)

CHAPTER 12

Musculoskeletal/injuries

MANAGING PAIN

OTC Analgesics

Guidance to CCGs from NHS England in 2018 stated that analgesics available over the counter (OTC) should not be prescribed for self-limiting musculoskeletal pain. Indeed, if the patient pays prescription charges, ibuprofen[P] and paracetamol are considerably cheaper if bought OTC. They may be used together up to their maximum daily doses although, curiously, the low-dose combination of paracetamol 500 mg plus ibuprofen 200 mg gave results that were almost as good as the higher doses, so perhaps this should be our first suggestion for acute pain (Table 12.1).

Paracetamol alone has no benefit over placebo in back pain or osteoarthritis (da Costa et al., 2017). Combination analgesics containing codeine[PBC] are available OTC, but to obtain additional analgesia from codeine[PBC], most people need to take at least 25 mg per dose, and many common combinations contain suboptimal doses. Suggest that the patient discusses this with the pharmacist. It should be noted that there is considerable individual variation in the response to non-steroidal anti-inflammatory drugs (NSAIDs) and opioids.

Taking analgesics with food substantially reduces their efficacy. Despite the commonly recommended advice to take analgesics with food, the evidence that this reduces adverse effects is non-existent (Rainsford 2012). Nor is there any evidence that rapidly dissolving formulations such as 'melts' are more effective or faster acting than ordinary tablets, but some compounds of ibuprofen are more rapidly absorbed into the bloodstream than others.

Table 12.1 Single dose pain relief after surgery

Medication	NNT for at least 50% pain relief
Ibuprofen acid 200	2.9
Ibuprofen acid 400	2.5
Ibuprofen fast acting[a] 200	2.1
Ibuprofen fast acting[a] 400	2.1
Diclofenac sodium 50	6.6
Naproxen 500	2.7
Ibuprofen 200 + paracetamol 500	**1.6**
Ibuprofen 400 + paracetamol 1000	**1.5**
Paracetamol 500	3.5
Paracetamol 1000	3.2
Paracetamol 1000 + codeine 60	2.2
Ibuprofen 400 + codeine 60	2.2
Codeine 60	12

Source: Moore, R. et al. 2015.
Lower number needed to treat (NNT) = better pain relief
[a] 'Fast-acting' refers to particular compounds of ibuprofen: lysine, arginine or sodium. These are available OTC or on prescription, but are significantly more expensive than ibuprofen acid.

There has been outcry surrounding the branding of some OTC medications, which may suggest targeted action against a particular cause of pain – that is, tension headache, period pain, migraine and back pain. Other than topical administration, there is no way of targeting the action of analgesia. Indeed, this type of branding can potentially be dangerous, with patients inadvertently overdosing through taking the same analgesic compound (but branded differently) repeatedly, that is, for their period pain, tension headache and back pain. An advert in the United Kingdom for Nurofen Joint and Back® was banned in 2016 for suggesting targeted pain relief, while in Australia, the manufacturer of Nurofen® was fined AUS$6 million in late 2016 for misleading consumers.

NSAIDs

- Contraindications to NSAIDs:
  - Allergy
  - Current peptic ulcer or GI bleed

- Renal failure (eGFR <30 mL/min)
- Liver failure
- Heart failure
- Inflammatory bowel disease
- Trying to conceive
- Pregnancy
- Naproxen[PBCI] is contraindicated if breastfeeding (ibuprofen[P] is the NSAID of choice if breastfeeding)
- Chickenpox or shingles
- Cardiovascular disease (Bally et al., 2017)
- Use NSAIDs with caution if:
  - Previous peptic ulcer or GI bleed
  - Male; GI bleed risk is twice as high in men
  - Older; GI bleed risk doubles with every decade above 55 years:
    - 1 per 1000 people per year at 55
    - 2 per 1000 people per year at 65
    - 4 per 1000 people per year at 75
  - Hypertension
  - Asthma (although most patients with asthma can take NSAIDs without a problem. Ask whether they have ever taken one before) (Kanabar et al., 2007)
  - Taking interacting medicines, for example, prednisolone, SSRIs, spironolactone, lithium
  - Within first 48 hours after surgery, fracture or injury (see Sprains section later in this chapter)
- NICE recommends co-prescribing a proton pump inhibitor (PPI – e.g. omeprazole[Q] 20 mg daily) to all patients over 45 given an NSAID for more than a short course, and it should be considered even for short courses if the patient is at high GI risk
- If one NSAID is ineffective, it is worth trying another, as there is considerable individual variation in response

Gabapentinoids

Gabapentin[PC] and pregabalin[PBC] are useful treatments for neuropathic (nerve damage) pain. This type of pain is recognised by its characteristics of feeling like electric shocks, stabbing, burning or cold, and it tends to radiate in narrow bands rather than being localised. Such pain often does not respond well to conventional analgesia (paracetamol, NSAIDs and opioids). The distinction between different types of pain is clinically important; for example, gabapentinoids may be helpful for treating sciatica but do not improve low back pain from strained ligaments or muscles.

There is increasing awareness that the gabapentinoids have significant potential for misuse, dependence and drug diversion. Pregabalin is likely to have a higher abuse potential due to its rapid absorption, faster onset of action and higher potency. Public Health England (2014) advises prescribers to inform patients of the risks of abuse and dependence, and that the rationale for prescribing decisions be discussed fully and documented. The Advisory Council on the Misuse of Drugs recommended to the government in 2016 that the drugs should be controlled as Class C substances. At the time of publication, this has not yet been implemented although it has been accepted in principle, subject to consultation.

The Medicines and Healthcare Products Regulatory Agency (MHRA) issued a drug safety update in October 2017 advising that gabapentin can cause respiratory depression, so caution needs to be taken if the patient is at increased risk (respiratory, neurological or renal disease, taking central nervous system depressants such as opiates or benzodiazepines, and the elderly).

Opioids

Opioids relieve pain by acting on endorphin receptors in the central nervous system (CNS) rather than tackling the cause of the pain; they have no anti-inflammatory action. Short-term use for musculoskeletal conditions may be needed if other analgesics fail to relieve pain, but beyond a 2-week course, dependency is a major risk and non-pharmacological treatments provide a far better option. In contrast to NSAIDs, where if a patient does not respond well to one, it is useful to try an alternative, the variation in response to opioids is more often related to genetic variations in the enzymes that metabolise opioids, rather than which opioid is used. The same dose of one opioid may give widely different therapeutic and adverse effects for different individuals. This is particularly true of tramadol, which is one reason why the National Minor Illness Centre (NMIC) does not encourage its use.

Codeine[PBC] is the most frequently prescribed opioid in the United Kingdom. Women in particular have variations in their metabolism of this opioid such that some convert 10% to morphine, while others convert 50%. As morphine is readily excreted into breast milk, this variation in metabolism prohibits the use of codeine in breastfeeding mothers. Children are very susceptible to adverse effects of morphine, so codeine is contraindicated for all children under 12 years and not needed for any minor illness for adolescents under 18 years. When required as a short course for adults, prescribe codeine separately from other analgesics such as paracetamol to allow flexibility in the dose and choice. When the pain is bad, the patient can take both drugs, and when pain starts to improve, the dose of codeine can be reduced first. As constipation is almost inevitable, always advise on a laxative (see section on Constipation in Chapter 9).

Chronic pain

- Defined as pain that has lasted for longer than 3 months after the usual recovery period for an illness or injury
- Although it can be felt in a specific part of the body (i.e. back, pelvis, abdomen), chronic pain may be a problem with the pain system itself rather than pathology in the area in which the pain is experienced
- While the World Health Organization (WHO) analgesic ladder was useful in guiding clinicians in controlling cancer pain, it is often inappropriately applied to the treatment of chronic pain
- Though analgesics are useful for acute pain, they are much less effective in chronic pain and can lead to more problems than benefits
- Opioids should not be used for chronic pain due to limited effectiveness and possible significant harm – this is reflected in the NICE guidance (2016) for low back pain and sciatica which states 'do not offer opioids for managing chronic low back pain'
- In addition to the commonly known side effects of opioids such as constipation, sedation and nausea, long term use can lead to impaired fertility, reduced libido, weight gain, depression and dependance. Pain levels may even increase through nervous system sensitisation
- Patients with chronic pain may worry that their pain indicates damage is occurring and therefore restrict their activities. It is important to reassure patients that this is not the case, and resuming normal activities where possible would be beneficial
- A biopsychosocial approach is required to help people with chronic pain. Particularly when there is no target for medical or surgical intervention, patients will need support to learn to live and cope with their pain – they should therefore be offered psychological support and may need referral to an ACT-based (acceptance and commitment therapy) pain management programme
- The self-help guide on MoodJuice for chronic pain is excellent. Direct patients to www.moodjuice.scot.nhs.uk/chronicpain.asp

References

Advisory Council on the Misuse of Drugs. 2016. Letter to the home office re gabapentin and pregabalin. www.gov.uk/government/uploads/system/uploads/attachment_data/file/491854/ACMD_Advice_-_Pregabalin_and_gabapentin.pdf.

Bally, M., Dendukuri, N., Rich, B., Nadeau, L., Helin-Salmivaara, A., Garbe, E., and Brophy, J. 2017. Risk of acute myocardial infarction with NSAIDs in real world use: Bayesian meta-analysis of individual patient data. *BMJ*; 357: j1909. *This huge observational study found that NSAIDs were associated with an increased risk of acute myocardial infarction of up to 50%, greatest during the first month of NSAID use and with higher doses. For this reason, NMIC believes that NSAIDs are contraindicated in all patients with cardiovascular disease despite the European Medicines Agency statement: www.ema.europa.eu/ema/index.jsp?curl=pages/medicines/human/referrals/Ibuprofen_and_dexibuprofen_containing_medicines/human_referral_prac_000045.jsp&mid=WC0b01ac05805c516f.*

da Costa Bruno, R., Reichenbach, S., Keller, N., Nartey, L., Wandel, S., Jüni, P., and Trelle, S. 2017. Effectiveness of non-steroidal anti-inflammatory drugs for the treatment of pain in knee and hip osteoarthritis: A network meta-analysis. *Lancet*; 390(10090): e21–33. http://dx.doi.org/10.1016/S0140-6736(17)31744-0

Dalton, S.O., Johansen, C., Mellemkjær, L., Sørensen, H.T., Nørgård, B., and Olsen, J.H. 2003. Use of selective serotonin reuptake inhibitors and risk of upper gastrointestinal tract bleeding: A population-based cohort study. *Arch Intern Med*; 163(1): 59–64.

Faculty of Pain Medicine. 2015. Core standards for Pain Management Services in the UK. www.rcoa.ac.uk/system/files/FPM-CSPMS-UK2015.pdf.

Kanabar, D., Dale, S., and Rawat, M. 2007. A review of ibuprofen and acetaminophen use in febrile children and the occurrence of asthma-related symptoms. *Clin Ther*; 29(12): 2716–23. *This literature review found a low risk for asthma-related morbidity associated with ibuprofen use in children and a possible protective and therapeutic effect compared with paracetamol.*

Koren, G., Cairns, J., Chitayat, D., Gaedigk, A., and Leeder, S.J. 2006. Pharmacogenetics of morphine poisoning in a breastfed neonate of a codeine-prescribed mother. *Lancet*; 368(9536): 704. doi: 10.1016/S0140-6736(06)69255-6.

Leppert, W., and Mikolajczak, P. 2011. Analgesic effects and assays of controlled-release tramadol and o-desmethyltramadol in cancer patients with pain. *Curr Pharm Biotechnol*; 12(2): 306–312. doi: 10.2174/138920111794295738. *The blood level of tramadol cannot be predicted by the dose. If there is no suitable alternative, start at a low dose and titrate carefully.*

MHRA Drug Safety Update. July 2013. Codeine for analgesia: Restricted use in children because of reports of morphine toxicity. www.gov.uk/drug-safety-update/codeine-for-analgesia-restricted-use-in-children-because-of-reports-of-morphine-toxicity.

MHRA Drug Safety Update. 26th October 2017. Gabapentin (Neurontin): Risk of severe respiratory depression. www.gov.uk/drug-safety-update/gabapentin-neurontin-risk-of-severe-respiratory-depression#reminder-of-risk-with-concomitant-use-of-opioids.

Moore, R., Derry, S., Aldington, D., and Wiffen, P. 2015. Single dose oral analgesics for acute postoperative pain in adults – an overview of Cochrane reviews. *Cochrane Database of Systematic Reviews*; (9). Art. No.: CD008659. doi: 10.1002/14651858.CD008659.pub3. *For single-dose pain relief after surgery.*

Moore, R., Derry, S., Straube, S., Ireson-Paine, J., and Wiffen, P. 2014. Faster, higher, stronger? Evidence for formulation and efficacy for ibuprofen in acute pain. *Pain*; 155(1): 14–21. www.ncbi.nlm.nih.gov/pubmed/23969325. doi: 10.1016/j.pain.2013.08.013. *Interesting reference suggesting that ibuprofen arginine, lysine and sodium salts are more effective than standard ibuprofen.*

Moore, R., Derry, S., Wiffen, P., and Straube, S. 2015. Effects of food on pharmacokinetics of immediate release oral formulations of aspirin, dipyrone, paracetamol and NSAIDs – a systematic review. *Br J Clin Pharmacol*; 80(3): 381–388. doi: 10.1111/bcp.12628. *There is evidence that high, early plasma concentrations produce better early pain relief, better overall pain relief, longer lasting pain relief and lower rates of re-medication. Taking analgesics with food may make them less effective, resulting in greater population exposure. It may be time to rethink research priorities and advice to professionals, patients and the public.*

NICE CKS. 2015. NSAIDs – prescribing issues. cks.nice.org.uk/nsaids-prescribing-issues.

NICE NG59. 2016. Low back pain and sciatica in over 16s: Assessment and management. www.nice.org.uk/guidance/NG59.

Petersen, J., Hallas, J., de Muckadell, O.B., Dall, M., and Hansen, J.M. 2014. A model to assess the risk for ASA/NSAID-related ulcer bleeding for the individual patient based on the number of risk factors. *Gastroenterology*; 146(5): S-319. www.gastrojournal.org/article/S0016-5085(14)61148-3/pdf.

Public Health England. 2014. Advice for prescribers on the risk of the misuse of pregabalin and gabapentin. www.gov.uk/government/uploads/system/uploads/attachment_data/file/385791/PHE-NHS_England_pregabalin_and_gabapentin_advice_Dec_2014.pdf.

Rainsford, K.D., and Bjarnason, I. 2012. NSAIDs: Take with food or after fasting? *Journal of Pharmacy and Pharmacology*; 64(4): 465–469. onlinelibrary.wiley.com/doi/10.1111/j.2042-7158.2011.01406.x/epdf.

NECK PAIN

History

- Patient concerns (meningitis?)
- Duration
- Injury, for example, whiplash
- Site of pain
- Fever
- Sore throat
- Occupation (e.g. checkout/keyboard operator)
- 🚩 Rheumatoid or inflammatory arthritis
- 🚩 Neurological symptoms

Examination

- Range of movement
- Location of pain (muscle or vertebra)
- If infection suspected:
  - Temperature, pulse rate and blood pressure
  - Cervical lymph nodes
  - Neck stiffness (can a child kiss his knees?)

Self-care

- Reassure about meningitis (if appropriate)
- Explain that neck pain is common and likely to resolve in 3–4 weeks
- Continue normal activity as much as possible

- Cervical collars are not recommended
- Sleep with one firm pillow
- Try to maintain good posture
- Consider workstation assessment
- Do not drive if neck movements are restricted
- Analgesia with ibuprofen[P]/paracetamol
- If pain is muscular, try diclofenac emulgel[PC]

RED FLAGS

- Neurological symptoms (*possible prolapsed cervical disc/myelopathy; seek urgent advice from a senior colleague*)
- Sudden-onset severe headache with neck stiffness (*possible subarachnoid haemorrhage; call 999*)
- Rheumatoid or inflammatory arthritis (*may affect the atlantoaxial joint, making it unstable. Refer same day to Rheumatology*)
- Localised tenderness over one vertebra (*may suggest metastasis or osteoporotic wedge fracture; refer to a senior colleague*)

References

Derry, S., Wiffen, P., Kalso, E., Bell, R., Aldington, D., Phillips, T., Gaskell, H., and Moore, R. 2017. Topical analgesics for acute and chronic pain in adults – an overview of Cochrane Reviews. *Cochrane Database of Systematic Reviews*; 5. Art. No.: CD008609. doi: 10.1002/14651858.CD008609.pub2. *There was good evidence that topical NSAIDs are useful in acute pain conditions such as sprains or strains. Different formulations varied in effectiveness; the best was diclofenac emulgel (NNT 1.8).*

NICE CKS. 2015. Neck pain – non-specific. cks.nice.org.uk/neck-pain-non-specific.

BACK PAIN

Most back pain is muscular; the differential diagnosis includes sciatica (about 10% of cases, due to pressure on nerve roots) and rare conditions such as spinal cord compression, spinal fracture, metastases, infection and spondyloarthritis.

History

- What is worrying you? (often prolonged debility)
- Onset: gradual/sudden/while lifting
- Duration
- Any previous episodes
- Site – make sure it really is in the back, not the kidney, lung or hip
- Radiation to leg – especially below the knee
- Numbness/tingling of each leg
- Weakness in any area, particularly movements of each leg
- Occupation
- Psychosocial stress
- Where are they sleeping (bed, sofa or floor?)
- ⚑ Difficulty passing urine
- ⚑ Disturbed sensation in perineum (wiping after going to the toilet may feel different/numb)
- ⚑ Abdominal pain/coldness/cyanosis of legs
- ⚑ Fever

🏴 Weight loss/malaise

🏴 Osteoporosis

🏴 Previous cancer/tuberculosis

🏴 Immunosuppressed/IV drug user

Examination

- Ask patient to show site of pain and palpate the area
- Spinal tenderness/scoliosis/abnormal shape
- Spasm of paraspinal muscles
- If leg symptoms, check straight leg raising – record angles

Tests

- Not necessary or helpful. Patients who expect an x-ray should be gently told that it will be of no help in finding the cause of their pain (unless fracture is suspected), and the dose of radiation required is 120 times that of a chest x-ray. MRI scans are generally not indicated either unless the patient is considering surgery, there are rapidly evolving neurological symptoms, or red-flag pathology is suspected. Most back pain is muscular, and no current scan can pinpoint this

Self-care

- Reassure the patient that most back pain, even with sciatica, is not serious and will get better without treatment. Pain does not equal damage
- Explain that stress causes muscular tension and can contribute to pain; relaxation or meditation may help
- Reducing movement may delay recovery, so encourage gentle mobilisation (activity within the limits of pain as soon as possible)
- Give exercise leaflet, for example, from Arthritis Research UK but explain (if appropriate) that their back pain is not caused by arthritis. (It is worth noting that Arthritis Research UK has many other excellent exercise leaflets)
- If mattress is over 10 years old, consider buying a new one
- Carefully applying heat to the area may be helpful
- For acute back pain, regular analgesics are recommended because they help the patient to keep mobile
- Manipulative therapies such as osteopathy and chiropractic are available privately (or through insurance schemes). NICE recommends that they should only be used in conjunction with an exercise regime
- Consider a TENS machine if symptoms persistent (although not recommended by the latest NICE guidance)
- The patient's emotional health plays a major part in the resolution of their back pain, and it is very important that health professionals convey a positive attitude from the beginning. The STarT Back tool may be used to identify patients who are at high risk of persistent symptoms – if so, *refer to Musculoskeletal Service*
- Cognitive-behavioural interventions such as the BeST programme are effective at reducing pain and disability at 12 months and improving patient satisfaction and quality of life
- See earlier section on Chronic pain if appropriate

Prescription

- If ibuprofen[P] OTC has been ineffective, consider naproxen[PBCI] (500 mg twice daily for adults)
- Codeine[PBC] may be prescribed separately from paracetamol as codeine phosphate[PBC] tablets (adult dose: initially 30 mg every 4 hours as required, increasing to 60 mg if necessary, maximum dose 240 mg per 24 hours) if necessary for acute pain. This is likely to cause constipation, which may be difficult to manage when the patient has back pain, so always offer a laxative (see section on Constipation in Chapter 9). Opioids should not be used for chronic low back pain
- If ordinary analgesics are ineffective, particularly if muscles are in spasm, a short course of diazepam[PB] (5 mg one to three times daily for adults) may be offered, but warn the patient about possible drowsiness and driving impairment
- For sciatica, if NSAIDs are ineffective or inappropriate, consider gabapentin[PC] (see earlier section on gabapentinoids). Pregabalin does not appear to be effective (Mathieson et al., 2017)

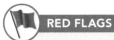

RED FLAGS

- Numbness/tingling in perianal area, bladder or bowel dysfunction (*possible cauda equina syndrome; urgently admit under Orthopaedics*)
- Sudden-onset severe back and abdominal pain, with discoloration of legs or stiffness (*possible dissection of aortic aneurysm; call 999*)
- Sudden-onset severe headache with back stiffness (*possible subarachnoid haemorrhage; call 999*)
- Osteoporosis or cancer patients (even if thought to be in remission) with sudden onset of severe pain over a vertebra, tender on examination and relieved by lying down (*possible spinal fracture/metastasis; discuss with senior colleague/Oncology*)
- New onset aged >50 years (*higher risk of osteoporotic fracture or cancer; refer to senior colleague*)
- Severe pain that remains when supine, night pain that disturbs sleep, or pain aggravated by straining (*possible metastatic cancer; refer to senior colleague*)
- Thoracic pain (*uncommon, higher risk of metastatic cancer; discuss with senior colleague*)
- Fever and malaise, especially in immunosuppressed patients, IV drug users or those with tuberculosis (*possible spinal infection; admit under Orthopaedics*)
- Weight loss (*may be undiagnosed cancer; refer to senior colleague*)

References

Keele University. 2011. STarT Back Tool. www.keele.ac.uk/sbst/startbacktool/.

Knox, C.R., Lall, R., Hansen, Z., and Lamb, S.E. 2014. Treatment compliance and effectiveness of a cognitive behavioural intervention for low back pain: A complier average causal effect approach to the BeST data set. *BMC Musculoskelet Disord*; 15(1): 17.

Mathieson, S., Maher, C.G., McLachlan, A.J., Latimer, J., Koes, B.W., Hancock, M.J., Harris, I. et al. 2017. Trial of pregabalin for acute and chronic sciatica. *New England Journal of Medicine*; 376(12): 1111–1120. *Treatment with pregabalin did not significantly reduce the intensity of leg pain associated with sciatica and did not significantly improve other outcomes.*

NICE NG59. 2016. Low back pain and sciatica in over 16s: Assessment and management. www.nice.org.uk/guidance/NG59.

SPRAINS AND STRAINS

A sprain is a stretch or tear of a ligament; a strain is a stretch or tear of a muscle.

History

- How and when did it happen?
- Severity of impact (may suggest likely consequences)
- Location of any pain and what makes it worse
- Timing of pain. Immediate pain and loss of function make fracture more likely, whereas delayed pain and swelling suggest soft tissue injury
- Relevant medical and drug history, particularly osteoporosis and anticoagulants
- Functional loss (e.g. weakness)
- Instability or 'giving way'
- Neurological symptoms
- Does anything make you suspect abuse?

Examination

- Swelling (note that this takes time to develop – in primary care, patients often present very early)
- Assess possibility of fracture/dislocation (see Box 12.1):
  - Degree of bruising
  - Any deformity
  - Bony tenderness

- Ability to weight bear, if relevant
- Restriction of movement. If passive movements are pain-free, then fracture is unlikely
- Assess circulation (warmth/pulses/capillary refill) and sensation distal to injury

---

BOX 12.1 INDICATIONS FOR X-RAY AFTER ACUTE INJURY (IF NOT OBVIOUS FRACTURE)

Ankle: pain over the malleolus AND *one of the following:*

- Inability to bear weight for at least four steps
- Bone tenderness along the distal 6 cm of the posterior edge of the fibula or tip of the lateral malleolus
- Bone tenderness along the distal 6 cm of the posterior edge of the tibia or tip of the medial malleolus

Foot: pain in the midfoot zone AND *one of the following:*

- Inability to bear weight for at least four steps
- Bone tenderness at base of the fifth metatarsal
- Bone tenderness of the navicular bone (distal to the medial malleolus)

Knee:

- Inability to bear weight for at least four steps
- Age 55 years or above
- Tenderness at the head of fibula
- Isolated tenderness of patella
- Inability to flex knee to 90 degrees

Wrist:

- Pain or tenderness over the scaphoid bone

Diagrams available online:

www.mdcalc.com/ottawa-ankle-rule.

www.ohri.ca/emerg/cdr/knee_formats.html.

Self-care

- Follow **PRICE** for 3 days after the injury:
  - **P**rotect from further injury
  - **R**est – avoid activity for 3 days and then mobilise
  - **I**ce (e.g. pack of frozen peas, wrapped in a towel to avoid skin damage)
  - **C**ompression (e.g. with Tubigrip) may relieve symptoms of joint injuries, except for the ankle where there is no evidence of benefit
  - **E**levation above the level of the heart
- Avoid **HARM** for 3 days:
  - **H**eat (e.g. hot baths, heat pads)
  - **A**lcohol (increases bleeding and swelling)
  - **R**unning (or other exercise)
  - **M**assage (may worsen bleeding and swelling)
- A short period of immobilization may speed recovery in strains and severe sprains
- Take paracetamol or use topical diclofenac emulgel[PC] for pain relief, but NSAIDs are not recommended in the first 48 hours because they may delay the healing process. Inflammation plays an important part in healing (NICE CKS, 2016)
- Opioids do not appear to be more effective in acute sprains and fractures than the combination of paracetamol and ibuprofen (at least at the doses conventionally used)

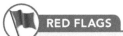
RED FLAGS

Refer same-day to Paediatrics/Orthopaedics if:

- Safeguarding concerns; any injury in a non-mobile child is suspicious (*it would be worth 'calling-ahead' and highlighting your concerns about possible non-accidental injury with the paediatric team before the child arrives at hospital*)
- Swelling of an area and known bleeding disorder (*e.g. swollen knee + haemophilia = possible haemarthrosis*)
- Inability to bear weight (walk four steps). Ankle sprains are often painful on initial walking and then improve
- Penetrating injury to joint
- Suspected:
  - Dislocation, complete muscle tear or complete tendon rupture (*deformity/instability/inability to perform certain movements*)
  - Damage to nerves or circulation
  - Septic arthritis (*fever with hot, red and swollen joint – may follow penetrating injury*)
  - Bleeding into joint (*very painful, rapid swelling*)
  - Fracture (*see Box 12.1*)

References

Bendahou, M., Khiami, F., Saïdi, K., Blanchard, C., Scepi, M., Riou, B., Besch, S., and Hausfater, P. 2014. Compression stockings in ankle sprain: A multicenter randomized study. *Am J Emerg Med*; 32(9): 1005–1010. www.researchgate.net/profile/Pierre_Hausfater/publication/263318576_Compression_Stockings_in_Ankle_Sprain_A_multicenter_Randomized_Study/links/54e212070cf2966637943dee.pdf. *Compression stockings did not improve the time to return to painless walking and delayed the return to sports.*

Chang, A.K., Bijur, P.E., Esses, D., Barnaby, D.P., and Baer, J. 2017. Effect of a single dose of oral opioid and nonopioid analgesics on acute extremity pain in the emergency department: A randomized clinical trial. *JAMA*; 318(17): 1661–1667. jamanetwork.com/journals/jama/article-abstract/2661581. *In this RCT of patients with limb pain following injury, there was little difference in the effects of various combinations of analgesics.*

Derry, S., Wiffen, P., Kalso, E., Bell, R., Aldington, D., Phillips, T., Gaskell, H., and Moore, R. 2017. Topical analgesics for acute and chronic pain in adults – An overview of Cochrane Reviews. *Cochrane Database Syst Rev*; (5): Art. No: CD008609. doi: 10.1002/14651858.CD008609.pub2. *There was good evidence that topical NSAIDs are useful in acute pain conditions such as sprains or strains. Different formulations varied in effectiveness; the best was diclofenac emulgel (NNT 1.8).*

NICE CKS. 2016. Sprains and strains. cks.nice.org.uk/sprains-and-strains.

van den Bekerom, M., Struijs, P., Blankevoort, L., Welling, L., Niek van Dijk, C., and Kerkhoffs, G. 2012. What is the evidence for rest, ice, compression, and elevation therapy in the treatment of ankle sprains in adults? *J Athl Train*; 47(4): 435–443. doi: 10.4085/1062-6050-47.4.14. *Good question. Answer: Not a lot.*

HEAD INJURY

History

- How did it happen?
- How long ago?
- Headache
- Neck pain
- Recent intake of alcohol or recreational drugs
- Loss of consciousness
- Vomiting since injury – particularly worrying if worsening
- Confusion, amnesia, drowsiness, convulsions
- Neurological disturbance (e.g. numbness, weakness, double vision)
- Blood or clear fluid from ear or nose

🚩 Bleeding disorder, anticoagulants

🚩 Does anything make you suspect abuse?

Examination

- Is the patient confused/drowsy? Assess using the Glasgow Coma Scale (see Box 12.2)
- Examine site of injury, look for and measure any bruising or swelling
- If examining a child under 2 years, check for a bulging fontanelle
- Check pupils:
  - Are they equal?
  - Do they react to light?
  - Any photophobia?

BOX 12.2 GLASGOW COMA SCALE (GCS) FOR ADULTS AND VERBAL CHILDREN

Best eye response:

- Does not open eyes – score 1
- Opens eyes in response to painful stimuli – score 2
- Opens eyes in response to voice – score 3
- Opens eyes spontaneously – score 4

Best verbal response:

- Makes no sounds – score 1
- Incomprehensible sounds – score 2
- Inappropriate words – score 3
- Confused and disorientated – score 4
- Orientated and converses normally – score 5

Best motor response:

- Makes no movement in response to pain – score 1
- Extension in response to painful stimuli – score 2
- Abnormal flexion in response to painful stimuli – score 3
- Flexion or withdrawal in response to painful stimuli – score 4
- Localises painful stimuli – score 5
- Obeys simple commands – score 6

Self-care for adults

- Rest as much as possible
- Take paracetamol, if needed, for headache
- If appropriate, inform employer about head injury and consider graded return to work
- Until completely recovered, avoid:
  - Being alone or out of telephone contact
  - Alcohol or sedative medicines
  - NSAIDs (for the first 2 days)
  - Contact sports
  - Driving or operating machinery
- Go to A&E immediately if:
  - Becoming drowsy or confused
  - Fluid leaks from the ear or nose
  - Bruising develops behind the ears
  - Developing problems with sight, understanding, memory or speech

- Develop loss of balance or weakness in arms or legs
- Headache gets worse
- Vomiting

Advice to parents about caring for children

- Offer paracetamol if required for headache
- Offer only light meals for 1 or 2 days
- Until completely recovered, **avoid**:
  - Leaving child alone. Check them every couple of hours while they are asleep (but do allow them to sleep; don't keep them awake)
  - Giving ibuprofen
  - Overexcitement
  - Contact sports and rough play
- If appropriate, inform teacher that child has had a head injury and consider graded return to school
- Go to A&E immediately if concerned or if child:
  - Becomes drowsy or confused
  - Leaks fluid leaks from ear or nose
  - Develops bruising behind the ears
  - Develops problems with sight, understanding, memory or speech
  - Develops loss of balance or weakness in arms or legs
  - Complains of worsening headache
  - Cries persistently
  - Vomits three or more times

RED FLAGS

Refer urgently to A&E or appropriate speciality if:

- High-energy impact to head, for example, fall from a height of >1 metre or >5 stairs
- GCS less than 15 (*i.e. any impairment*)
- Any history of loss of consciousness
- Amnesia lasting more than 5 minutes
- Confusion, convulsions or any other neurological disturbance
- Vomiting (*more than once in an adult or ≥3 in a child*)
- Persistent and worsening headache
- Bleeding disorder or taking anticoagulant
- Previous brain surgery
- Intoxication
- Suspicion of a non-accidental injury (*e.g. non-mobile child, inadequate explanation, delayed presentation, other injuries, previous safeguarding concerns*)
- In children under 2 years, a bulging fontanelle – indicating raised intracranial pressures (*the anterior fontanelle has generally closed by 2 years of age*)
- In children under 1 year, a bruise, swelling or laceration of more than 5 cm on the head
- Suspected skull fracture (*periorbital haematoma without local injury, deafness, clear cerebrospinal fluid from ear or nose, bleeding from ear, bruising behind ear*)
- Pupils unequal or non-reactive, or photophobia

Consider sending the patient to hospital for monitoring if there is no one to supervise them at home, even if the red flag criteria are not met.

Reference

NICE CG176. 2017. Head injury: Assessment and early management. www.nice.org.uk/guidance/cg176.

JOINT PAINS

Arthralgia is common; patients may be concerned that they have developed rheumatoid arthritis. Here is a brief overview:

- Shoulder pain: younger adults may suffer from dislocations or disorders of the acromioclavicular joint. In people aged 30–60, pain is most likely to be due to rotator cuff tendinopathy or a 'frozen shoulder'; over the age of 60, osteoarthritis becomes more likely
- Elbow pain in an adult is most likely to be tennis elbow
- Knee pain in adolescents may be due to Osgood-Schlatter disease. In young adults, patellofemoral pain syndrome is common; in older adults, suspect osteoarthritis
- Hip pain in older patients is most likely to be due to osteoarthritis or greater trochanteric pain syndrome. Beware hip pain and limp in children (slipped femoral epiphysis, Perthes' disease)
- Thumb and finger pain is usually due to osteoarthritis
- Toe pain is usually caused by gout if it occurs episodically

Osteoarthritis is a common joint disorder that mostly affects the knees, hips and small joints of the hands. It is more common with increasing age, but may also affect people in their 40s. The joints are not hot or swollen but are painful when used; there may be crepitus or restriction of movement. Pain tends to be worse after activity or at the end of the day. Diagnostic tests such as x-rays are only useful if surgery is being considered and do not always correlate with clinical severity.

Rheumatoid arthritis (RA) usually starts with inflammation affecting the small joints of the hands and the feet. It affects 1% of the population and is commoner in women in their 40s and 50s. The key features are swelling, heat and pain in the affected joints, often with stiffness after inactivity. Morning stiffness lasting at least 30 minutes is suggestive, and symptoms are usually symmetrical. All patients suspected of having RA should be referred for specialist assessment; blood tests (e.g. rheumatoid factor, ESR) are unreliable. Other types of inflammatory arthritis include systemic lupus erythematosus, psoriatic arthritis and ankylosing spondylitis.

References

Gray, M., Wallace, A., and Aldridge, S. 2016. Assessment of shoulder pain for non-specialists. *BMJ*; 355: i5783. doi.org/10.1136/bmj.i5783.
Red Whale. 2018. Lateral hip pain and greater trochanteric pain syndrome. www.gp-update.co.uk/SM4/Mutable/Uploads/pdf_file/Lateral-hip-pain-and-greater-trochanteric-pain-syndrome.pdf

GOUT

This disorder of purine metabolism is more common in men aged 30–60. Due to high levels of uric acid in the blood, crystals form in the cooler areas of the body, typically the first metatarsophalangeal joint (at the base of the great toe) but also in tophi (swellings often found on the elbow or pinna).

History

- Location of pain
- Speed of onset (often rapid, within 24 hours)
- Previous episodes and response to treatment
- Diet – particularly offal, game, oily fish, seafood and meat/yeast extracts (Bovril or Marmite)
- Alcohol intake
- Medication – aspirin, diuretics
- ⚑ Any fever/malaise

Examination

- Temperature and pulse rate (fever or tachycardia would suggest possible septic arthritis)
- The joint is swollen, hot, red and painful on passive movement with gout. May affect any joint, more commonly the lower limb, and often not symmetrical. Over time, attacks of gout can involve multiple joints at once
- Tophi – firm white nodules on pinnae, elbows, fingers, toes or knees. Usually occur when gout is long-standing

Tests

- Serum uric acid measurement may help the diagnosis, but
  - Should be delayed until at least 4 weeks after the attack, and

- False-positives and false-negatives are common
- If the diagnosis is uncertain, consider testing ESR, rheumatoid factor and anti-nuclear antibodies

Self-care

- Rest and elevate the limb
- Use an ice pack, for example, frozen peas wrapped in a towel
- Drink plenty of water
- Reduce alcohol intake – particularly beer and spirits
- Reduce consumption of sugars, especially fructose
- Reduce consumption of liver, kidneys, red meat, oily fish, yeast extracts, seafood and certain vegetables (asparagus, beans, cauliflower, lentils, mushrooms and spinach)
- Vitamin C supplements have been recommended, but the evidence is not convincing
- A helpful diet sheet is available from the UK Gout Society – www.ukgoutsociety.org/docs/goutsociety-allaboutgoutanddiet-0113.pdf

Action

- First-line treatment is naproxen[PBCI] (for adults, initially 750 mg, then 250 mg every 8 hours until attack has passed). Note that patients with gout are often at increased cardiovascular risk
- If NSAIDs are not suitable, prescribe colchicine[PCI] (for adults, 500 mcg 2–4 times a day until symptoms are relieved, maximum 6 mg per course; do not repeat course within 3 days) or prednisolone (for adults, 30 mg daily for 5 days). An unfortunate side effect of colchicine is diarrhoea – not ideal when mobilizing is painful
- Intra-articular corticosteroid injections may be used if oral treatment is unsuitable or ineffective
- People with frequent episodes of gout, or with tophi, may be offered prophylaxis with allopurinol[PCI]. It takes 2–3 months to work, during which time an NSAID or colchicine should be co-prescribed, and urate levels should be monitored

 RED FLAG

- Pain, heat and swelling in a single joint associated with fever or malaise (*suspect septic arthritis; admit under Orthopaedics*)

References

Jamnik, J., Rehman, S., Blanco Mejia, S., de Souza, R., Khan, T., Leiter, L., Wolever, T., Kendall, C., Jenkins, D., and Sievenpiper, J. 2016. Fructose intake and risk of gout and hyperuricemia: A systematic review and meta-analysis of prospective cohort studies. *BMJ Open*; 6(10): e013191. doi: 10.1136/bmjopen-2016–013191. *Fructose consumption was associated with an increased risk (62%) of developing gout in predominantly white health professionals.*

NICE CKS. 2015. Gout. cks.nice.org.uk/gout.

Stamp, L., O'Donnell, J., Frampton, C., Drake, J., Zhang, M., and Chapman, P. 2013. Clinically insignificant effect of supplemental vitamin C on serum urate in patients with gout: A pilot randomized controlled trial. *Arthritis & Rheumatism*; 65: 1636–1642. doi: 10.1002/art.37925. *Vitamin C (500 mg/day) for 8 weeks had no clinically significant urate-lowering effects in patients with gout.*

ROAD TRAFFIC COLLISION – ASSESSMENT

Be aware that patients may present for a wider range of reasons than simply concern over their symptoms; they may think it important that they attend to justify a future claim for compensation, or they have been advised to be 'checked over' by the police or an insurance company. The first doctor to provide emergency treatment after a road traffic accident is entitled to charge a fee of £21.30: see www.bma.org.uk/advice/employment/fees/emergency-treatment.

History

- Date and time of the collision
- Were they the driver or a passenger/a pedestrian/a cyclist?
- Details of the collision – how did it happen, were they moving or stationary?
- Direction of impact
- If in a car, whether passenger or driver, if a seat belt was worn, whether there was a head restraint and if air bags were activated

- Descriptions of the injuries: pain, stiffness, bruising, and so forth
- If neck pain, was it immediate with restricted movement, or delayed?
- Psychological effects: shaking, insomnia, nightmares, fear of driving, flashbacks (important for compensation)
- Time off work/school
- 🚩 Any functional loss (e.g. weakness)
- 🚩 Instability or 'giving way'
- 🚩 Disturbance of bladder/bowel function or perianal numbness

Examination

- Appropriate to affected area
- Extent of grazing and bruising – measure these
- Movement of affected limbs or neck – check for any limitation of range
- Assess possibility of fracture/dislocation (see Box 12.1)

Action

- Give treatment and advice dependent on, and appropriate to, the injuries
- Sketch areas of grazing and bruising, or recommend a police photograph
- Often the main purpose of the patient's visit is to document the injuries for a possible future compensation claim. Record the details carefully

RED FLAGS

- Any suspicion of fracture or dislocation (see Box 12.1) (*refer same day to Orthopaedics*)
- Any suspicion of spinal cord or cauda equina compromise – weakness in limbs, loss of sensation, disturbance of bladder or bowel function, perianal numbness (*urgently admit under Orthopaedics*)

BITES – ANIMAL AND HUMAN

History

- Which part of the body?
- How did it happen?
- Which animal? (Note that the answer may not be truthful, especially with human bites)
- Date/time of bite
- Did it happen abroad?
- Any fever or feeling unwell?
- 🚩 Is there a background of:
  - Immunosuppression
  - Structural heart disease
  - Prosthetic joint
- 🚩 Does anything make you suspect abuse/any safeguarding concerns?

Examination

- Temperature and pulse rate
- Look for cellulitis – is the surrounding area hot, red and tender?
- Is there discharge from the wound?
- How deep is the wound?
- Any teeth or foreign bodies in the wound?

Tests

- Consider wound swab

Self-care

- Check for signs of infection, and if these develop, seek help immediately
- For bite on leg, elevate the leg

Action

- If fresh wound, irrigate with warm water
- If possible, remove any foreign bodies (such as teeth) from the wound
- Consider need for vaccination against tetanus and hepatitis B
- Consider post-exposure prophylaxis against rabies and HIV
- Consider antibiotic (Box 12.3)

 BOX 12.3 ANTIBIOTICS FOR ANIMAL AND HUMAN BITES

Give antibiotics if:

- Human or cat bite less than 3 days old
- Affecting the hand, foot or face
- Puncture wound
- Possible bone or joint penetration
- Immunosuppressed
- Prosthetic joint
- Artificial heart valve

Antibiotic choice in adults

- Co-amoxiclav (500/125 mg three times daily for 7 days)
- If allergic to penicillin:
    - Human bites: use a 7-day course of clarithromycin[PIQ] 500 mg twice daily plus metronidazole[Q] 400 mg three times daily
    - Animal bites: use a 7-day course of doxycycline[PBC] 100 mg twice daily plus metronidazole[Q] 400 mg three times daily
    - Review in 1–2 days as not all pathogens are covered by the alternatives to penicillin

 RED FLAGS

- Risk of rabies, for example bat bite (*phone Virus Reference Dept. of Public Health England on 020 8327 6017 to obtain rabies immunoglobulin*)
- Risk of hepatitis B or HIV (*seek specialist advice*)
- *Refer urgently to relevant specialty if:*
    - Penetrating wound affecting deeper structures
    - Bites to poorly vascularised areas, for example, ear or nose
    - Facial wounds (unless very minor) or scalp bite in a child
    - Suspected foreign body in wound or in need of closure
    - High risk group: immunosuppressed, severe liver disease, prosthetic valve or joint
    - Severe cellulitis/infected wounds not responding to treatment/systemically unwell
    - Safeguarding concerns, for example, human or dog bite to a child

References

Aziz, H., Rhee, P., Pandit, V., Tang, A., Gries, L., and Joseph, B. 2015. The current concepts in management of animal (dog, cat, snake, scorpion) and human bite wounds. *Journal of Trauma and Acute Care Surgery*; 78(3), 641–648. http://s3.amazonaws.com/academia.edu.documents/44628839/The_current_concepts_in_management_of_an20160411–4533-1ecyphu.pdf?AWSAccessKey Id=AKIAIWOWYYGZ2Y53UL3A&Expires=1501254769&Signature=hdUZ4eacbfmjtV5nSUwYejoiYak%3D&response-content-disposition=inline%3B%20filename%3DThe_current_concepts_in_management_of_an.pdf. *The use of prophylactic antibiotics in dog bites should be limited to patients who have a high risk of infection.*

NICE CKS. 2015. Bites – Human and animal. cks.nice.org.uk/bites-human-and-animal.

INSECT BITES AND STINGS

There is a temptation to overtreat insect bites or stings with antibiotics because the appearance of the normal inflammatory response to the sting toxin may look like an infection. In fact, very few bites in the United Kingdom become infected. If the bite was sustained abroad, record the details carefully in case the patient presents later with symptoms that could be a disease from the bite, such as malaria or leishmaniasis.

History

- Site
- Time of bite/sting, if known
- Nature of insect, if known
- Itching
- Previous severe reaction to bites (suggests allergy)
- Generalised rash
- Fever/general malaise
- ⚑ Breathing difficulty

Examination

- Temperature and pulse rate
- Size of reaction
- Evidence of lymphangitis or cellulitis
- Is sting still in situ (rare)

Self-care

- Except for jellyfish stings, wash area with soap and water and apply ice pack to reduce swelling
- For jellyfish stings, wash in vinegar and apply a hot pack for 40 minutes
- Try not to scratch – consider brushing with a clean paintbrush to reduce itching without damaging the skin
- Take an oral antihistamine, for example, loratadine (10 mg once daily for adults)
- If still itching, consider adding oral chlorphenamine[PBI] (4 mg for adults) at night, if sedation tolerated
- Evidence is lacking for topical applications
- Piezo-electric devices may reduce itching; they are available OTC for around £7
- Seek help urgently if developing breathing difficulty
- Seek help if becoming feverish or signs of infection developing
- Seek help if rash develops after tick bites (could be Lyme disease; see Box 12.4)

Action

- If stinger still in place, remove it as soon as possible by scraping with a scalpel blade, not tweezers
- Remove ticks as soon as possible. Specialist tick removers are available; otherwise, tweezers may be used. Heat, Vaseline® and alcohol are not recommended. Warn about signs of Lyme disease (Box 12.4)
- It may sometimes be difficult to distinguish the expected normal inflammatory response or allergy from infection. Allergic reactions usually occur within the first 24 hours. Signs of infection usually develop after 24 hours, with increasing redness, tenderness and swelling. Other signs may include:
  - Fever
  - Pus
  - Lymphangitis (tracking)

Prescription

- If infection is suspected, treat with flucloxacillin (500 mg four times daily for adults) or, if allergic to penicillin, clarithromycin[PIQ] (500 mg twice daily for adults). A delayed prescription may be appropriate
- If still itching, consider adding oral ranitidine (150 mg twice daily for adults – *unlicensed indication*)
- Severe local reactions may require oral prednisolone[IP] (40 mg once daily for adults), but do not prescribe if possibly infected

---

BOX 12.4 LYME DISEASE

A bacterial infection carried by deer ticks. Cases occur mainly in forested areas. The risk is low if the tick has been attached for less than 24 hours, but people do not always notice the tick.

A round spreading red area develops around the site of the bite, typically one week later, and spreads; usually larger than 5cm with central clearing. It may be painful or itchy, and the person may feel unwell with flu-like symptoms.

Laboratory tests are available, but are not necessary if the classical rash of erythema migrans is present (NICE, 2018).

If diagnosis is likely, treat adults with doxycycline[PBC] 100mg twice daily for 21 days.

 RED FLAGS

Call 999 if:

- Swelling of lips or tongue
- Breathing difficulty
- Anaphylactic shock (*extremely rare*)

References

Doyle, T., Headlam, J., Wilcox, C., MacLoughlin, E., and Yanagihara, A. 2017. Evaluation of Cyanea capillata. Sting management protocols using ex vivo and in vitro envenomation models. *Toxins*; 9: 215. www.mdpi.com/2072-6651/9/7/215. After a sting by a lion's mane jellyfish (the most common UK type), washing in vinegar and applying a hot pack for 40 minutes was the most effective treatment.

NICE CKS. 2016. Insect bites and stings. cks.nice.org.uk/insect-bites-and-stings.

NICE NG95. 2018. Lyme disease. www.nice.org.uk/guidance/ng95.

Public Health England. 2014. Suggested referral pathway for patients with symptoms related to Lyme disease. webarchive.nationalarchives. gov.uk/20140714085912/ www.hpa.org.uk/webc/HPAwebFile/HPAweb_C/1317141297288.

SUNBURN

History

- Country and duration of exposure
- Sunscreen usage
- Fluid intake and urine output
- Any safeguarding concerns

Examination

- Temperature
- Extent of burn
- Redness
- Blistering
- Skin loss

Self-care

- Cool the skin by having a cool shower or bath; do not apply ice
- Drink plenty of cool fluids
- Avoid alcohol
- Apply emollient or aloe vera gel (only to intact skin)
- Leave blisters intact if possible
- Apply non-adherent dressings, for example, Jelonet® to areas of skin loss

Caution

- If temperature is elevated, assess level of hydration, and treat for heatstroke with rest, fluids and cooling

References

Genuino, G., Baluyut-Angeles, K., Espiritu, A., Lapitan, M., and Buckley, B. 2014. Topical petrolatum gel alone versus topical silver sulfadiazine with standard gauze dressings for the treatment of superficial partial thickness burns in adults: A randomized controlled trial. *Burns*; 40(7): 1267–1273. www.sciencedirect.com/science/article/pii/S0305417914002526. *Petrolatum gel without top dressings may be at least as effective as silver sulfadiazine gauze dressings in the treatment of minor superficial partial thickness burns in adults.*

Harding, M. 2015. Sunburn. patient.info/doctor/sunburn.

BURNS AND SCALDS

A burn is caused by heat or electricity, whereas a scald is caused by hot liquid or steam. Superficial burns or partial-thickness burns covering less than 5% of the body are called minor burns.

History

- Parts of body affected
- Cause of burn/scald
- How it occurred and duration of contact
- What has been done so far?
- Is it painful? (Full-thickness burns are not painful)
- ⚑ Any safeguarding concerns

Examination

- Check temperature and pulse rate – evidence of sepsis?
- Extent of burn – how many palmprints of the patient is the size of the burn?
- Depth of burn is assessed through colour change/vesicles/capillary refill (tested using sterile cotton bud or swab)
    - Superficial epidermal burns are red but not blistered. Capillary refill – blanches and refills rapidly
    - Partial thickness – superficial dermal burns are pale pink with blistering. Capillary refill – blanches and refills slowly
    - Partial thickness – deep dermal burns are blotchy and red with possible blistering. Capillary refill – does not blanch
    - Full-thickness burns look leathery or waxy. The skin may be white, brown or black with no blisters. Capillary refill – does not blanch
- In dark skin, superficial or partial thickness may not appear red
- Evidence of possible inhalation injury (burnt nasal hairs, carbon in sputum)

Self-care

- Ensure safety (e.g. from flames, chemicals or electricity)
- Irrigate the burn as soon as possible with cool or tepid water, by immersing the area for between 10 and 30 minutes. Do not use iced water
- Keep the person warm to avoid hypothermia if cooling large areas
- If swollen, elevate the affected limb
- Take paracetamol for pain relief
- Apply emollients two to three times daily
- If referring to hospital (see section that follows), cover the burn with cling film, but do not wrap it all round the limb. Use a clean, clear plastic bag for hands or feet

Action

- Clean area with sodium chloride 0.9% or lukewarm tap water
- Consider aspirating any vesicles/bullae that are likely to burst; otherwise leave them intact
- If blistered, cover with a non-adherent dressing (e.g. paraffin gauze – Jelonet®) then a dressing pad and bandage. Review after 48 hours

- See Red Flags section that follows for all people who need referral to hospital. Also consider referral for:
  - Superficial dermal burns
  - Children under 5 years
  - Adults over 60 years
  - People with co-morbidities/immunosuppressed/pregnant
  - Social reasons, pain control or if dressings difficult to manage

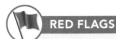

RED FLAGS

Admit under Medical/Paediatrics/Plastic Surgery if:
- Signs of infection/sepsis/systemically unwell
- Safeguarding concerns
- All deep dermal and full-thickness burns
- Burn goes completely around the body or a limb
- Area larger than two palmprints in a child under 16
- Area larger than three palmprints in an adult
- Involving the face, hands, feet, perineum, genitalia or any flexure
- Any electrical, cold or chemical burn
- Any inhalation injury

Refer any burn that has not healed after 2 weeks to a specialist burn unit.

References

National Burn Care Referral Guidance. 2012. www.webarchive.org.uk/wayback/archive/20130325152202/www.specialisedservices.nhs.uk/library/35/National_Burn_Care_Referral_Guidance.pdf.
NICE CKS. 2015. Burns and scalds. cks.nice.org.uk/burns-and-scalds.

LACERATIONS/WOUND INFECTIONS

Assess the risk of infection (e.g. contamination, co-morbidities, immunosuppression) and check for signs of sepsis, if relevant.

History
- Wound location
- How did it occur?
- How long ago did it happen?
- Has the wound been contaminated?
- Immunosuppression/diabetes
- Any safeguarding concerns

Examination
- Check temperature and pulse rate
- Is there evidence of infection?
- Wound length
- Wound margins – are they jagged?
- Is there any contamination?

Self-care
- Disinfect the skin with antiseptic, but try not to get it into the wound
- Remove any foreign bodies, under local anaesthetic if necessary
- Take paracetamol for pain relief
- Seek help if increasing pain/redness/swelling or fever/malaise

Action

- Irrigate with sodium chloride 0.9% solution
- Assess risk of infection – high risk would be wound contamination or two or more of the following (although use your clinical judgement):
  - Age over than 65 years
  - Wound length more than 5 cm
  - Jagged wound margin
  - Immunosuppression/diabetes
  - Injury more than 6 hours ago
- Consider closure only if no signs of infection and low risk:
  - Tissue glue, self-adhesive strips or both, can be used to close wounds less than 5 cm where the edges can be easily pulled together. This is not practical near the eye (where glue could seriously damage the surface), for areas that cannot be covered by a dressing to stop them getting wet (when adhesives will fail), or on a joint (unless it is going to be immobilised for at least 5 days)
  - Suturing: for wounds not suitable for closure with glue or self-adhesive strips (see above)
  - Strips/sutures can be removed after 3–5 days for head wounds, 10–14 days for wounds over joints, 7–10 days for other sites
- Dress with a clear vapour-permeable dressing; use an absorbent pad if exudate is present
- Check tetanus immunisation status and offer immediate booster if needed (response may take up to 7 days; the incubation period for tetanus is 4–21 days. See Public Health England, 2018)
- If a tetanus-prone wound occurs in a patient who has not had five tetanus vaccinations (with the last dose within 10 years), tetanus immunoglobulin may be indicated, although it is in short supply (Public Health England, 2018)
- If infected, take a swab and prescribe flucloxacillin (500 mg four times daily for adults) or, if allergic to penicillin, clarithromycin[PIQ] (500 mg twice daily for adults). If wound contaminated with high-risk material, instead use co-amoxiclav (500/125 mg three times daily for adults)
- For infected wounds after surgery, take a swab and contact the responsible surgeon (ideally before prescribing, although this may not be practical)
- If high risk for infection but no features of current infection, consider prophylactic antibiotics
- If wound not closed initially due to infection/high infection risk, review in 3–5 days to see if wound can be closed

RED FLAGS

Admit under Medical/Paediatrics/Orthopaedics/Plastic Surgery if:

- Signs of sepsis
- High risk of tetanus
- Safeguarding concern
- Damage to bone, artery, nerve or tendon
- Facial laceration
- Signs of infection of the hand, face or near a joint

References

Aresti, N., Kassam, J., Bartlett, D., and Kutty, S. 2017. Primary care management of postoperative shoulder, hip and knee arthroplasty. *BMJ*; 359: j4431. doi.org/10.1136/bmj.j4431. *Do not treat suspected wound infections empirically with antibiotics without advice from the operating surgeon, as it may diminish the ability to later isolate an organism to treat.*

McVicar, J. 2013. Should we test for tetanus immunity in all emergency department patients with wounds? *Emerg Med J*; 30: 177–179.

NICE CKS. 2017. Lacerations. cks.nice.org.uk/lacerations.

Public Health England, 2018. Recommendations on the treatment and prophylaxis of tetanus. https://assets.publishing.service.gov.uk/government/uploads/system/uploads/attachment_data/file/728172/Recommendations_on_the_treatment_and_prophylaxis_of_tetanus_July2018.pdf

CHAPTER 13

Management of minor illness

EVIDENCE-BASED PRACTICE

Evidence-based practice is 'the integration of the best available evidence with our clinical expertise and our patients' unique values and circumstances'. It is helpful for all clinicians working in primary care to be consistent and evidence-based in managing minor illness. Where differences in practice are apparent, you should be able to access up-to-date, high-quality research evidence to aid discussion and help you to reach agreement. Critical analysis of published research has become highly complex and very time consuming; thankfully, there are now several agencies such as the Cochrane Collaboration that analyse the evidence on your behalf and provide easy access to this information on the Internet.

Although these reviews explore possible flaws in the published papers, there are several factors that inherently bias the whole process of evaluating evidence. They include:

- Old drugs may appear inadequately researched compared to new ones
- Large samples are needed to compare one intervention with another reliably, but this can obscure the benefit or harm to a smaller group of people, with a particular characteristic, who form just part of that larger group
- Participants in research trials are often highly selected; they may be healthy or have just the one disease requiring the treatment being researched, whereas, in practice, patients often have several diseases and may be taking many drugs
- There are some physiological differences between different populations (hence the differential management of blood pressure). The population evaluated in a trial may not reflect the patient in front of you
- Trials on new medicines are too short to pick up long-term side effects – this must come later from monitoring
- When real outcomes are too infrequent to be examined, surrogate measures are used (e.g. serum cholesterol as opposed to death from heart attack), but these may not reflect the true outcome
- Few trials examine the whole patient: an antihypertensive may reduce the risk of stroke, but did it cause more falls or road traffic accidents due to faintness?
- The rigorous standards and large sample sizes that are now expected in clinical trials lead to very high costs, which make it difficult to attract funding other than from pharmaceutical companies with a high turnover
- Funded research is more likely to favour the sponsor's product
- Negative results are less likely to be published
- Little research is conducted in primary care
- Therapies that do not employ the same disease categories as Western medicine are almost impossible to research using randomised controlled trials
- Many established therapies do not have a good evidence base because it would be unethical to withhold them for trial purposes. 'No evidence of effectiveness' is not the same as 'evidence of non-effectiveness'

What we call 'evidence' is an artificial construction, a man-made concept that should not be confused with truth. Patients will have a very different perspective to clinicians on what factors would persuade them to try a new therapy. Bearing these limitations in mind, it is important to recognise that guidance needs to be placed in the context of your patient's situation. The more experienced you become, the more confidence you will have to deviate from standard advice and target treatment to the individual needs of a patient; it is important that your reasons are documented.

We recommend the following resources:

- NICE CKS: cks.nice.org.uk (excellent, evidence-based, practical guidance). The recommendations given here were extensively checked against Clinical Knowledge Summaries (CKS) guidance at the time of writing
- NHS Evidence: www.evidence.nhs.uk. An Athens password is needed to access some of the resources; those working in the National Health Service (NHS) can obtain this by registering on the site
- Cochrane library: www.cochranelibrary.com. A huge database of systematic reviews
- Trip database: www.tripdatabase.com for the answer to that awkward question

HOLISTIC CARE

It is apparent from reading the other chapters of this book that the previous optimism of Western medicine about the eradication of infectious diseases through antibiotics has not been fulfilled. The more that we research these drugs, the more evidence we find that their benefits in most cases of minor illness are marginal, yet little evidence exists to support alternative treatments (including traditional self-care advice about rest and fluids) nor is such evidence likely to be provided because funding for research into minor illness and the relief of self-limiting symptoms remains limited.

You may feel that this lack of evidence-based treatments leaves you in an awkward position; the patient is coming to you for help, and you have little to offer. Your priority must be to establish that there is no indication of serious disease and, if so, to reassure the patient accordingly and give appropriate 'worsening advice'. It is important to be sensitive to their ideas, concerns and expectations, or 'agenda'. They may have attended to legitimise their illness to an employer or at the insistence of a relative. Social factors, such as an impending holiday or examination, are often of far greater importance to people than any medical issues and can inevitably influence their assessment of the relative risks and benefits of any treatment. Patients often attend for reassurance and do not necessarily want advice on managing their illness. Furthermore, offering unsolicited advice on treatment may encourage the patient to come back the next time they have the same self-limiting symptoms, which is wasteful for the health service and creates a culture of dependency.

In Western medicine, the 'placebo effect' is regarded as a nuisance that interferes with the evaluation of the 'real' effects of a treatment in clinical trials, yet the placebo effect is itself very real and enhances the intrinsic healing ability of the body (curiously this may happen even if people are aware that they are taking a placebo – seen in so-called 'open label placebo' trials). You can harness this effect very easily by establishing a good relationship with the patient, being positive and emphasising that a good recovery is likely. The placebo effect of any treatment that you suggest will be enhanced by the fact that you have recommended it. If you recommend a treatment that does not have a good evidence base, you need to use your clinical judgement as to how to share this information with the patient (which will inevitably reduce the effectiveness). It is also clearly inappropriate to recommend such a treatment if there is a risk that it may do harm.

References

Ballou, S., Kaptchuk, T.J., Hirsch, W., Nee, J., Iturrino, J., Hall, K.T., Kelley, J.M. et al. 2017. Open-label versus double-blind placebo treatment in irritable bowel syndrome: Study protocol for a randomized controlled trial. *Trials*; 18: 234. doi.org/10.1186/s13063-017-1964-x. *A review of open-label placebo treatment.*

Gabbay, J., and le May, A. 2016. Mindlines: Making sense of evidence in practice. *BJGP*; 66(649): 402–403. bjgp.org/content/66/649/402. doi: 10.3399/bjgp16X686221. *'Coffee-room chat may impact on evidence-based practice at least as much as all those guidelines'.*

Greenhalgh, T., Howick, J., and Maskrey, N. 2014. Evidence based medicine: A movement in crisis? *BMJ*; 348: g3725. doi: 10.1136/bmj.g3725. *A thorough critique of evidence-based medicine.*

Jefferson, T., and Jørgensen, L. 2018. Redefining the 'E' in EBM. *BMJ Evidence-Based Medicine*; 23: 46–47. doi.org/10.1136/bmjebm-2018-110918. *Wonderful quote: 'By the law of Garbage In Garbage Out, whatever we produce in our reviews will be systematically assembled and synthesised garbage with a nice Cochrane logo on it'.*

Resnick, B. 2017. The weird power of the placebo effect, explained. *Vox.* www.vox.com/science-and-health/2017/7/7/15792188/placebo-effect-explained. *A very clear explanation of the complex mechanisms though which placebos work and the new ways of using them. 'Placebo is … the water that medicine swims in'.*

MAKING A DIAGNOSIS

The skills needed to make a diagnosis take time to acquire. Experienced clinicians tend to diagnose by 'pattern matching' – a few pointers will lead them quickly to the most likely possibility. The working diagnosis often starts at a very early stage – even when you are reviewing the patient's notes before calling them into the room. It may be changed by your observation of their behaviour and appearance in the waiting room or in the corridor, then change again with their first sentence. Information that is volunteered spontaneously by the patient is much more likely to be relevant than that acquired by asking direct questions. This 'working diagnosis' process is usually efficient, but it has some pitfalls; jumping to the wrong conclusion is the most obvious. In order to reduce this risk, it is wise to ask yourself three questions:

- Is there anything that does not fit with this diagnosis?
- What other diagnoses are possible?
- Am I confident that the management of this situation is within my boundaries of expertise and clinical practice?

REMOTE ASSESSMENT

Through the National Minor Illness Centre's courses, we have encountered some confusion amongst attendees about whether it is appropriate for an independent prescriber to prescribe for a patient following a consultation by telephone or online. There is nothing in the regulations to prevent this; the Nursing & Midwifery Council (NMC) has issued specific guidance about remote prescribing, which states 'you must satisfy yourself that you have undertaken a full assessment of the patient/client, including taking a full history and, where possible, accessing a full clinical record'. A face-to-face consultation or physical examination may be helpful to establish a diagnosis but is not mandatory. An example of a diagnosis when a remote consultation would provide adequate assessment is uncomplicated cystitis, which can be diagnosed and treated based on a good history.

Reference

NMC. 2015. Practice Standard 20 in standards of proficiency for nurse and midwife prescribers. uk/globalassets/sitedocuments/circulars/2008circulars/nmc-circular-16_2008.pdf.

ARE THERE ANY TYPES OF PATIENTS THAT YOU SHOULD NOT SEE?

Clinicians come to minor illness management from a wide range of backgrounds, and it is not possible to make blanket recommendations. It is more efficient for you to exclude patients with issues that you are unable to resolve, such as someone requesting a second or third opinion for a complex chronic problem. Paediatricians sometimes recommend that only clinicians with a paediatric qualification should see children; this is simply impractical and would exclude many General Practitioners (GPs). It is sometimes also suggested that only those with a midwifery qualification should see pregnant women. This is not only impractical but also potentially dangerous, resulting in 'de-skilled' clinicians failing to consider pregnancy in a pregnant female who is unaware. The Royal College of Nursing (RCN) provides the following guidance for independent prescribers: *'A useful distinction may be whether the "condition" is related to the pregnancy or not; even then we would recommend consideration of the possible impact on pregnancy and consult appropriately'*. If there are several clinicians within an organisation who see patients with minor illness and they all have different exclusions, it becomes a logistical nightmare to book patients with the appropriate person.

Reference

Royal College of Nursing. 2017. Prescribing in pregnancy: The role of independent and supplementary nurse prescribers. www.rcn.org.uk/clinical-topics/medicines-optimisation/specialist-areas/prescribing-in-pregnancy.

CHILDREN

The examination of children requires a child-friendly environment and special skills: See *Spotting the Sick Child* (reference follows).

- Bring your face to their level
- Keeping your voice soft, explain what you want to do but do not explicitly ask their permission. The parent/guardian has already given their implied consent
- Talk about something of interest to them
- Encourage parent to cuddle them
- Non-threatening examination first – for example, hands
- Then chest, in case the child cries later
- With an anxious or uncooperative child, first listen to the chest through thin clothes, then undress the child and listen again
- If the child is crying by then, listen carefully during inspiration
- Leave throat until last, and only examine if necessary
- Firm hold is needed for ear examination to avoid hurting the child if they wriggle

All clinicians working with children should be aware of current advice on Safeguarding Children and should have undergone training to Level 3. This can be accessed through your local Safeguarding Children Board and may be available online.

References

HM Government. 2015. Working together to safeguard children. www.gov.uk/government/publications/working-together-to-safeguard-children--2. *Statutory guidance on inter-agency working to safeguard and promote the welfare of children.*
www.spottingthesickchild.com. *An excellent free resource with learning materials on the signs and symptoms of serious illness in children.*

INFECTIONS

The traditional Western explanation of the infectious process portrays the human body as a sterile environment that has been invaded by a hostile organism. Our scientists' efforts have been concentrated on finding newer and better chemical weapons to defeat these enemy forces. However, the spread of antibiotic resistance is causing increasing concern. Our ability to develop new antibiotics is limited; all antibiotics in our formulary were developed more than 30 years ago.

We are beginning to see that this warlike model is fundamentally flawed. The human body is more like an ecosystem, supporting a myriad of other organisms far greater in number than the cells in our body. Some of them are essential for our survival and exist with us in symbiosis, such as the intestinal bacteria that manufacture vitamin K. Broad-spectrum antibiotics dramatically alter our internal flora, leading to side effects such as diarrhoea and vaginal thrush.

Many of the organisms that can cause infections are normal inhabitants of the healthy human body (*commensals*) (Table 13.1). The process that causes them to become pathogenic is not well understood, but it often seems to be initiated by a fall in the vigilance of the immune system rather than a change in the organism itself. The immune system has intricate links with all other systems of the body, is in communication with the gut bacteria, and is susceptible to the effects of nutrition and psychosocial stress. It follows from this that the maintenance of a healthy body and mind is important, both in reducing the chances of developing an infection and in aiding recovery. It also seems logical that medicines that interfere with the natural defences of the body (e.g. anti-pyretic, anti-emetic and anti-inflammatory drugs) should be used with caution.

Table 13.1 Some of the bacteria that cause common infections and the antibiotics most frequently used against them

Organism	Commensal	Diseases	Antibiotic susceptibility
Streptococcus	Throat	Pharyngitis, otitis media, pneumonia, meningitis, cellulitis	**Phenoxymethylpenicillin**, amoxicillin, clarithromycin[PIQ]
Staphylococcus	Nose	Impetigo, boils, abscesses, cellulitis	**Flucloxacillin**, clarithromycin[PIQ]
Haemophilus influenzae	Upper respiratory tract	Otitis media, epiglottitis, meningitis, chest infections	**Amoxicillin** (80%), co-amoxiclav, clarithromycin[PIQ], doxycycline[PBC]
Escherichia coli	Intestine	UTI, abscesses, gastro-enteritis	**Nitrofurantoin**[PBC*] (97%), trimethoprim[PI] (71%), cefalexin, pivmecillinam[P]

Main source: Public Health England. 2017. AMR local indicators. fingertips.phe.org.uk/profile/amr-local-indicators. *Local and national antibiotic resistance figures*
* Nitrofurantoin should only be used for lower UTI because blood and tissue levels are low.

Recurrent infections

Sometimes a patient presents with several different types of infection over a short period of time. Consider if they are in a high-risk group for infections (see Chapter 2). If there is no apparent reason for the recurrences, there may be an underlying problem (see Box 13.1).

BOX 13.1 HIDDEN CAUSES OF RECURRENT INFECTIONS

- Increased exposure to infections (e.g. child starting school)
- Psychosocial stress (*a potent immunosuppressant for viral infection*)
- White cell dysfunction (*e.g. leukaemia – check full blood count*)
- Undiagnosed diabetes (*check fasting plasma glucose or HbA1c if appropriate; see Box 8.2 (Checking for Diabetes) in Chapter 8*)
- Human immunodeficiency virus (*HIV; offer testing*)
- Immunoglobulin deficiency, in children and young people (*check FBC and immunoglobulin levels*)

References

Blaser, M.J. 2014. The microbiome revolution. *J Clinical Invest*; 124(10): 4162–4165. www.jci.org/articles/view/78366. doi: 10.1172/JCI78366. *An overview of new approaches to the microorganisms that live in and on the human body. For the full story, see the author's book Missing Microbes 2015 ISBN-13: 978–1250069276.*

Pedersen, A., Zachariae, R., and Bovbjerg, D. 2010. Influence of psychosocial stress on upper respiratory infections – A meta-analysis of prospective studies. *Psychosomatic Medicine*; 72(8): 823–832. journals.lww.com/psychosomaticmedicine/Abstract/2010/10000/Influence_of_Psychological_Stress_on_Upper.14.aspx. doi: 10.1097/PSY.0b013e3181f1d003. *Still the best review of the evidence for the effects of stress on immunity.*

Public Health England. 2017. AMR local indicators. fingertips.phe.org.uk/profile/amr-local-indicators. *Local and national antibiotic resistance figures.*

Thaiss, C.A., Zmora, N., Levy, M., and Elinav, E. 2016. The microbiome and innate immunity. *Nature*; 535(7610): 65–74. www.nature.com/nature/journal/v535/n7610/full/nature18847.html?foxtrotcallback=true. doi: 10.1038/nature18847. *The intestinal microbiome is a signaling hub that integrates environmental inputs, such as diet, with genetic and immune signals to affect the host's metabolism, immunity and response to infection.*

NOTIFIABLE DISEASES

Diseases that must be notified to the local Health Protection Team (HPT) include:

- Suspected food poisoning (not in Scotland)
- Measles
- Mumps
- Rubella
- Pertussis
- Scarlet fever (in England and Northern Ireland)
- Chickenpox (only in Northern Ireland)

Full lists for each of the four UK countries and contact details of local HPTs are given on the websites below. This notification is statutory and does not require the patient's consent. Warn the patient that he or she may be contacted by the local HPT and explain that their role is to identify the source of infection and prevent its spread. If there are any implications for the community, for example, suspected food poisoning in a chef or a rare infectious disease, notify the local consultant in communicable disease by telephone. Information about specific diseases is given in Table 13.2.

LISTS OF NOTIFIABLE DISEASES

England: www.gov.uk/guidance/notifiable-diseases-and-causative-organisms-how-to-report#list-of-notifiable-diseases

Wales: www.wales.nhs.uk/sites3/page.cfm?orgid=457&pid=48544

Northern Ireland: www.niinfectioncontrolmanual.net/notifiable-diseases

Scotland: www.legislation.gov.uk/asp/2008/5/schedule/1

Table 13.2 Infectiousness and exclusion periods for various infectious diseases

Disease	Incubation period	Infective period	Exclusion from school/work	Action for contacts
Chickenpox	11–20 days	From 2 days before onset of rash to 5 days after	Until all vesicles are crusted (usually 5 days after rash appears)	Refer babies under 4 weeks old and non-immune immunosuppressed or pregnant contacts
Conjunctivitis	3–29 days	While discharge present	None	None
Cryptosporidium	2–5 days	While diarrhoea lasts	Until 48 hr after last diarrhoea or vomiting episode. No swimming for 2 weeks	HPT will decide
Diarrhoea and vomiting	1 hour–14 days (depending on cause)	While diarrhoea lasts	Until 48 hr after last diarrhoea or vomiting episode	No exclusion unless bacterial cause, when HPT will decide
Glandular fever	33–49 days	Variable	None	None
Hand, foot and mouth disease	3–5 days	Up to 7 days	None	None
Head lice	7–10 days	As long as lice or live eggs are present	None	None

(Continued)

Table 13.2 (*Continued*) Infectiousness and exclusion periods for various infectious diseases

Disease	Incubation period	Infective period	Exclusion from school/work	Action for contacts
Impetigo	1–10 days	While purulent lesions persist	Until lesions crusted, or 48 hr after treatment started	None
Measles	6–19 days	From 4 days before onset of rash to 4 days after	4 days from onset of rash	Refer babies under one year and non-immune immunosuppressed or pregnant contacts
Mumps	15–24 days	From 6 days before onset of symptoms to 4 days after	5 days from onset of swelling	None
Parvovirus (slapped cheek)	13–18 days	Until rash appears	None	Refer pregnant contacts under 30 weeks gestation
Pertussis (whooping cough)	5–21 days	Up to 3 weeks if untreated	Until 2 days after starting antibiotic, or 3 weeks after onset of symptoms if no antibiotic given	Consult HPT
Rubella (now very rare in UK)	13–21 days	From 13 days before onset of rash to 6 days after	4 days from onset of rash	Refer non-immune pregnant contacts under 20 weeks gestation
Scabies	7–27 days	Until mites and eggs have been destroyed	Until first treatment done	None once treated
Scarlet fever	12 hours–5 days	Up to 24 hr after antibiotic	24 hr after starting antibiotic treatment	None
Shingles	Not relevant	Until 5 days after onset of rash	None, provided lesions covered	Refer babies under 4 weeks and non-immune immunosuppressed or pregnant contacts if exposed to uncovered lesions
Threadworms	2–6 weeks	As long as eggs present	None	None once treated
Tinea	1–2 weeks	While lesions are active	None	None
Verrucas (plantar warts)	1–24 months	As long as warts are present	None (but cover warts with waterproof plaster for swimming/barefoot sports)	None

Main source: Public Health England (2018b and 2018c).

References

ECDC. 2016. Systematic review on the incubation and infectiousness/shedding period of communicable diseases in children. ecdc.europa. eu/sites/portal/files/media/en/publications/Publications/systematic-review-incubation-period-shedding-children.pdf. *Discusses the variation in advice about incubation and infectiousness from different sources.*

Medical Defence Union. 2017. Medico-legal guide to confidentiality: Notifiable infectious disease. www.themdu.com/guidance-and-advice/guides/confidentiality/notifiable-infectious-disease.

Public Health England. 2016. Rash in pregnancy. www.gov.uk/government/publications/viral-rash-in-pregnancy.

Public Health England. 2018a. Guidelines for the Public Health Management of Pertussis in England. https://assets.publishing.service. gov.uk/government/uploads/system/uploads/attachment_data/file/704482/Guidelines_for_the_public_health_management_of_ pertussis_in_England.pdf

Public Health England. 2018b. Health protection in schools and other childcare facilities. www.gov.uk/government/publications/ health-protection-in-schools-and-other-childcare-facilities.

Public Health England. 2018c. Infectious diseases A–Z. www.gov.uk/topic/health-protection/infectious-diseases.

CERTIFICATES

NHS certificates (fit notes, MED3s)

- May be used to state that the patient is unfit for any work
- Alternatively, the patient may be certified fit for limited work:
  - Phased return
  - Altered hours
  - Amended duties
  - Workplace adaptations
  - Other (in 'comments' box), for example, time off to attend appointments
- These should not be issued for the first 7 days of an illness. Employees who have been unwell for 4 or more days should obtain a Self-Certification (SC2) form from their employer or download one (just type SC2 into a search engine)
- Do not require face-to-face assessment
- May be completed after telephone consultation
- May be based on a written report by another registered healthcare professional (e.g. computer entry by minor illness nurse or pharmacist, or fax from an urgent care centre)
- Choice of 'open' statements (this will be the case for…) and 'closed' statements (from… to…)
- Use closed statements for most minor illness:
  - If the period is less than 14 days, and
  - The patient does not need to be reassessed
- Cannot be forward dated, although overlapping is permitted
- Closed statements can be backdated
- Those unable to claim statutory sick pay, such as self-employed people, may be eligible for Employment and Support Allowance or Universal Credit

Private certificates

These can be issued by GP practices at their discretion. There is a fee, which should be reclaimed from the employer. There is no need to supply sick notes for children's exams.

References

BMA. 2018. Childrens' exams. bma.org.uk/support-at-work/gp-practices/service-provision/supporting-pupils-at-school.

Citizens' Advice. 2018. www.citizensadvice.org.uk/work/rights-at-work/sick-pay/check-if-youre-entitled-to-sick-pay/.

Department for Work and Pensions. 2013. Fit note. www.gov.uk/government/collections/fit-note.

CHAPTER 14

Prescribing for minor illness

The range of medication required to treat minor illness found in this manual is limited to just over 100 commonly used medicines. Recommended indications and doses are given in the management section of each condition. To prescribe safely, you need to be aware of the action, side effects, interactions and contra-indications of each drug. Up-to-date information on each of these is available online in the British National Formulary (BNF), British National Formulary for Children (BNFC) (bnf.nice.org.uk) and the Summary of Product Characteristics (SmPC) (www.medicines.org.uk). Independent prescribers should be familiar with all these medicines already, but this alone is not enough to ensure safe practice. A sound knowledge of pharmacology and how drugs interact is essential because so many patients will be taking other medication. Furthermore, side effects of long-term medication are so common that about 1 in 30 consultations are because of symptoms masquerading as illness which are, in fact, caused by a medication. For this fifth edition of the manual, there is a new section on how to recognise adverse effects of commonly prescribed medication that can present as symptoms of minor illness. Elderly people, who have the greatest burden of medication, are at greatest risk.

PRESCRIBING SAFELY

Above all, make sure the prescription specifies the drug you intended. Most prescriptions in primary care are computer-printed. The difference between drugs with similarly spelt names can be as little as the gap between two adjacent keys on a keyboard used to select a drug from a list. One of the most dangerous examples is selecting penicillamine when penicillin was intended. Such an inadvertent swap from an antibiotic to an immunosuppressant could be fatal. It may seem that such a gross error is unlikely, but none of us is immune.

In 2004, the Royal College of General Practitioners, in collaboration with other national professional healthcare organisations and universities, sent their newsletter on prescribing entitled 'In Safer Hands' to all 9265 GP practices in England and Wales. The edition focused on different drugs with similar names. 'We have tried to make suggestions for redesigning systems to make medicines safer; however, as you will see, there is often no substitute for checking.' Next came a list of nine pairs of drugs most commonly confused with one another. Out of the 18 drug names, three were incorrectly spelt in the newsletter. This error rate of 1 in 6 is rather more than the average error rate in clinical practice of 1 in 20, as found in the PRACtICe Study (Avery et al., 2012).

As a final check before giving a prescription, the acronym *PASS* can be used to check if the patient is *pregnant, allergic*, on *something else* or has a *system failure*. When considering if a patient is pregnant, bear in mind those hoping to become pregnant but who have not yet missed a period; mothers who are breastfeeding also need caution when prescribing. Always check for interaction with any other current medication. Some drugs are contraindicated (i.e. should not be used) or should be given at lower dosage for patients with kidney, liver or heart failure. Information on this is given in the individual drug entries in the BNF. If in doubt, ask an experienced prescriber.

If you do need to write a prescription by hand, be aware of some additional pitfalls. The prescription form has a box at the top where the number of days' treatment may be entered. This avoids the need to calculate quantities but is awkward to use. It cannot be used for variable-dose drugs, creams, lotions, and so forth. Remember that the box is an instruction to the pharmacist as to how much to dispense, not a direction to the patient, so it does not appear on the dispensed medication instructions unless repeated in the main body of the prescription. It is simpler and clearer to specify an amount to be dispensed in the main text and leave the top box blank.

Clear, uncluttered prescriptions are safest. Try to avoid decimal points (e.g. 500 mg is preferable to 0.5 g), repeating words, using superfluous words (e.g. 'spoonful') or adding instructions that are on the medication label anyway. The wording of the cautionary and advisory label for any drug is to be found in the medicinal forms of the drug in the BNF online or book (referenced in the book to a list on the last page), or the medicines section of the app. As any required label is on the dispensed medication by default, there is no need to repeat it on a prescription. A different instruction can be added to a prescription if required, but it is best to avoid adding specific instructions when none are required, in case you inadvertently contradict the standard advice on how the medicine should be taken.

ABSORPTION

Not surprisingly, tablets and capsules are designed to dissolve very fast in the warm acid environment of the stomach. There is no need to prescribe liquid or dispersible medication to speed up absorption. Solid preparations are preferable, being chemically more stable and less expensive. Even in acute migraine, when the stomach may be immobile, the average difference in speed of absorption between tablets and liquid is only 10 minutes. Some tablets dissolve on the tongue (e.g. 'melts'), but the resulting liquid still needs to be swallowed. This is not for speed of onset, but when ordinary tablets cannot be swallowed easily, for example, when there is no ready access to water. There are very few preparations designed to be absorbed directly from the mouth, such as buccal prochlorperazine.

Modified-release tablets are designed to dissolve slowly to give a prolonged effect or reduced side effects. Gastro-resistant or enteric coating is a way of protecting a drug from damage by gastric acid. The coating resists acid but dissolves in the more alkaline small bowel, the main site of absorption of almost all oral drugs. Note that the coating is most often required to protect the drug, and only for a few medications is it helpful in protecting the patient's stomach. Gastric side effects are usually due to the overall effect of a drug after it has been absorbed, so the route by which it is given is immaterial. A non-steroidal anti-inflammatory drug can cause a gastric bleed from its systemic action, whether it is given orally, rectally or by injection.

Gastro-resistant coating overcomes a problem but introduces new ones for the prescriber. For example, 70%–90% of a dose of erythromycin is destroyed by normal gastric acid (Boggiano and Gleeson, 1976). Now consider the doses of erythromycin recommended in the BNF for different ages, which are all four times daily: 2–8 years 250 mg, doubled in more severe infections; 8–17 years 250–500 mg, doubled in more severe infection; and adult 250–500 mg, doubled in more severe infection. Can you see why the children's doses are so similar to the adult doses? There is a hidden assumption here that children will be prescribed a liquid form of the medicine, whereas adults are likely to have a gastro-resistant form that preserves the dose swallowed. This has implications for prescribers. A child who objects to the taste of a liquid medicine might prefer a solid form, but the use of a gastro-resistant form can result in a considerable increase in the effective dose absorbed. An adult with pneumonia who is allergic to penicillin might be prescribed erythromycin as an alternative, but beware that if they find it difficult to swallow capsules or tablets, a switch to a liquid preparation could reduce the absorbed dose to 10%–30% of what was intended. Trying to compensate for this by prescribing a higher dose would be fraught with difficulty because the amount of acid present when any one dose is swallowed might vary.

An added problem is that if an entire tablet or capsule is protected from dissolving in gastric acid, then the onset of action following the dose is delayed until the intact tablet or capsule happens to be near the opening pylorus, allowing passage into the duodenum and then on to the small bowel, the main site of absorption.

The conclusion for prescribers is to avoid gastro-protective coating when possible. If there is no form listed in the BNF without such coating, such as for omeprazole, or if most preparations that are listed are coated, then it may be necessary, but if there are many forms listed without gastro-protective coating, such as for prednisolone, or an alternative medication is available that is stable in acid, such as clarithromycin instead of erythromycin, then it is simpler and safer to use the uncoated option.

HALF-LIFE ($t_{1/2}$)

The speed at which a drug is eliminated from the body is usually proportional to the concentration of drug in the blood. Elimination is more rapid after a dose, when the drug is present in high concentration, than later when it is present only in low concentration. Drugs that are eliminated in proportion to their concentration are said to have first-order kinetics, and they have a constant $t_{1/2}$. This is the time taken for the concentration of the drug to reduce to one-half its starting level. Drugs with more complex kinetics may not have a constant $t_{1/2}$, but if it varies within a reasonably narrow range, then an average can be taken for practical purposes. It is useful to know the $t_{1/2}$, even if it is only an approximation, to help understand how long the action of a drug will last and when a further dose may be needed. This information may be found at www.medicines.org.uk by typing in the drug name, opening up the relevent SmPC and looking in Section 5.2. Although knowledge of $t_{1/2}$ is often helpful, some drugs have actions that last longer than the presence of the drug in the circulation; for example, the antiplatelet action of aspirin.

For a few drugs, the elimination rate stays constant because the metabolism for deactivating or eliminating it become saturated. Any further rise in the concentration of the drug in the blood does not drive faster elimination, as the process simply cannot go any faster. The maximum rate of ethanol metabolism is about one unit (10 ml) per hour, whether a single glass or a whole bottle of wine has been consumed. Regular consumption induces an increase in the speed of the enzymes up to the point when hepatic damage starts to impair the system.

ALLERGIES

Many reported allergies are just coincidences, for example, the appearance of a viral rash just after starting a course of an antibiotic. However, any report of swelling of the tongue or face, or difficulty in breathing, must be taken seriously.

Allergic reactions are usually:

- Itchy
- Generalised

- Confluent
- Either immediate (within 1 hour – often a more serious reaction) or occur 6–10 days after the drug is taken for the first time, or about 3 days after subsequent times, sometimes later

If the patient has a true allergy to one type of penicillin, *all* drugs of this class should be avoided. This does not apply if the patient experiences non-allergic side effects, such as diarrhoea with co-amoxiclav; phenoxymethylpenicillin may not produce this side effect. If penicillin is the first-line treatment but cannot be used because of a known penicillin sensitivity, the usual alternative is clarithromycin because it is a macrolide of very different structure to penicillin, and the spectrum of activity is similar. However, this too may be undesirable in view of its drug interactions. Azithromycin helps to overcome this problem, but both drugs are not recommended in pregnancy or for patients with a long QT interval. For further information, see the sections on *Prescribing in Pregnancy* and *QT Interval*. Cefalexin is the final alternative and can be used for patients sensitive to penicillin unless they have had an anaphylactic reaction to penicillin previously.

ADVERSE DRUG REACTIONS

Adverse drug reactions (ADRs), often referred to as 'side effects', are very common and becoming more so with increasing prescribing to prevent or control long-term conditions. A meta-analysis of hospital admissions between 1988–2015 showed that, for older people, 8.7% of hospital admissions resulted from an adverse reaction to medication (Oscanoa et al., 2017). We found no recent research into the impact of such reactions on primary care consultations, but our experience at the National Minor Illness Centre is that, in about 1 in 30 consultations, the presenting symptom is a result of an unwanted effect of medication. This equates to about one a day for a specialist clinician in minor illness. Thus, it is essential to consider acute symptoms in light of concurrent medication. If an ADR is suspected, the principle to follow is that it is far better to stop or change a medication that is causing problems than start another to control the unwanted effects. However, this is not always possible. If you do not normally prescribe the medication in question, seek advice from a clinician who does.

BOX 14.1 CLASSIFICATION OF ADVERSE DRUG REACTIONS

Two basic types:

    A. **A**ugmented (80%) (adverse amplified therapeutic effect)
    B. **B**izarre (20%) (but how could I have known that would happen?)

These can be divided into:

    C. **C**ontinuous (occurs while the drug is being taken)
    D. **D**elayed (occurs sometime after starting the drug)
    E. **E**nd of use (starts after the drug has been discontinued)

It may help in structuring your thoughts about ADRs to divide them into different types (Box 14.1).
One example of a drug that has the potential for an ADR in every one of these categories is prednisolone.

A. It is an immunosuppressant, but therapeutic effect increases the risk of infection.

B. Psychotic symptoms can be triggered; nothing to do with the therapeutic intention.

C. Immunosuppression continues while the drug is being taken.

D. Skin atrophy only occurs later if the drug is continued.

E. Stopping suddenly after prolonged use could precipitate an adrenal crisis.

DISCUSSING 'SIDE EFFECTS'

The debate over how much to say about side effects continues, with advocates at each end of the spectrum – from the view that one should say as little as possible for fear that otherwise the patient might not take the necessary treatment, to those who champion the notion that every possible side effect should be fully discussed. We must discount these extremes for what they are. The best way to encourage patients to take treatment when they really do need it is to involve them in the decision. It helps to have a background of not prescribing unnecessary treatment for them in the past. Always warn patients about important or common side effects, or any that are particularly relevant to them. Such a conversation may give you an insight into how much more information they would like to be given. Too little leaves them feeling uninformed and perhaps more vulnerable if problems do occur, and too much may cause unnecessary concern and confusion. Imagine trying to discuss fully the possible side effects of trimethoprim with the parents of a 3-year-old child with a proven urinary tract infection, namely that the antibiotic might cause toxic epidermal necrolysis or aseptic meningitis. Such serious side effects are vanishingly rare, but from the parents' point of view, it is difficult to appreciate the balance between the tiny risk involved and the essential need for treatment. The information leaflets that are provided with drugs rarely give the frequency of side effects, so very rare and serious ones may appear in a list together with common side effects that amount to no more than a nuisance.

It is the middle road for us – somewhere between the two extremes. It depends on your consultation skills exactly how well you manage to inform the patient about their proposed treatment. The aim is to give the patient any information that they either need or want. Always give instructions on how to take a medicine, even if it is on the prescription and will be duplicated on the label. If asked, 'Are there any side-effects?', the answer should be along the lines of 'Yes, all drugs have side effects, including this one', followed by an invitation to the patient to hear more about the specific side effects associated with the proposed treatment. Aim to cover everything the patient needs to know, and provide an easy opening for them to ask about anything they want to know as well. The BNF provides lists of known adverse reactions, but for more information or frequencies, look up the patient information leaflet or the more technical SmPC (www.medicines.org.uk/emc/). For antibiotic treatment, a study on hospitalised patients concluded that 1 in 5 would experience an adverse reaction (Tamma et al., 2017).

ADVERSE DRUG REACTIONS PRESENTING AS SYMPTOMS OF MINOR ILLNESS

Many drugs are used in primary care, and each one may have multiple adverse effects, so it is always worth considering if symptoms could be due to a drug rather than a new illness. Table 14.1 gives some of the more common ones. Unless you are an independent prescriber or have another specialist role, you may not be initiating these medications, but as a specialist in minor illness, it is important to recognise symptoms that might result from the patient's medication. Often the symptoms start shortly after starting a medication or changing the dose, but remember that type D adverse reactions are delayed.

Table 14.1 Symptoms which may be adverse reactions to medication

Adverse reaction symptom	Causative medication
Abdominal pain	Mebendazole, PPIs (e.g. omeprazole)
Arthralgia (gout)	Thiazides (e.g. bendroflumethiazide), aspirin
Confusion (hypoglycaemia)	Oral hypoglycaemics (e.g. gliclazide), insulin
Confusion (elderly)	Chlorphenamine, anticholinergics
Constipation	Opioids, PPIs, iron
Cough	ACE inhibitors (e.g. lisinopril)
Diarrhoea	Metformin, broad-spectrum antibiotics, laxatives, PPIs, colchicine, orlistat
Drowsiness	Sedative antihistamines (e.g. chlorphenamine), antiepileptics (e.g. carbamazepine, gabapentin, pregabalin, topiramate), opioids, benzodiazepines
Dyspepsia	NSAIDs including aspirin, bisphosphonates (e.g. alendronic acid), corticosteroids (e.g. prednisolone)
Eye pain (glaucoma)	Anticholinergics (e.g. ipratropium/tiotropium inhaler, doxazosin, amitriptyline, fluoxetine, citalopram), prednisolone
Fever	Meningitis B vaccine
Flushing	Tamoxifen
Headache	Analgesia overuse/withdrawal, CCBs (e.g. amlodipine), nitrates (e.g. isosorbide mononitrate), PPIs
Lightheadedness	Antihypertensives (e.g. doxazosin), diuretics (e.g. furosemide), sudden withdrawal of prednisolone
Myalgia	Statins (e.g. simvastatin) – *but rarer than patients think*
Nausea / vomiting	Colchicine, opioids, PPIs, metronidazole, nitrofurantoin, erythromycin, initial few weeks of SSRI (e.g. fluoxetine)
Petechiae	Antiplatelet drugs (e.g. aspirin), anticoagulants (e.g. warfarin), corticosteroids
Photosensitive skin	Tetracyclines (e.g. doxycycline)
Rash	Many drugs (e.g. penicillin, allopurinol)
Sore mouth (oral thrush)	Corticosteroid inhalers
Sore throat (urgent FBC needed)	Carbimazole, propylthiouracil, immunosuppressants
Swollen ankles	CCBs (e.g. amlodipine), corticosteroids (e.g. prednisolone)
Tremor / cramp / muscular spasm	Metoclopramide, prochlorperazine
Urinary frequency	Diuretics, SGLT2 inhibitors for diabetes (e.g. dapagliflozin)
Urinary retention	Chlorphenamine, anticholinergics
Wheezing	Beta-blockers (e.g. propranolol), NSAIDs

QT INTERVAL

A long interval between the Q and T waves on an electrocardiogram (ECG) indicates an increased risk of cardiac arrhythmias that can cause sudden death. People who inherit this characteristic should avoid all drugs that prolong the interval. Those who acquire it, by taking a drug that prolongs the interval, need to avoid taking a second drug that also prolongs the interval, thereby increasing the risk. The responsibility for this rests with the prescriber because most patients are unaware that they may be taking a drug that affects the QT interval. Anyone with a family history of unexplained sudden death should have an ECG, but if this has not been done before they need a medication, it would be wise to assume they might have an inherited long QT interval and avoid any drug that prolongs it.

Full information on which drugs prolong the QT interval can be found at the Sudden Arrhythmic Death Syndrome (SADS) website (www.sads.org.uk) or the American site CredibleMeds (www.crediblemeds.org). Below is a list of medications commonly prescribed in primary care or available over the counter (OTC) in the United Kingdom that are known to affect the QT interval. Not all carry the same risk. The drugs in bold type are associated with higher risk (Table 14.2).

Table 14.2 Common drugs that affect the QT interval (bold type indicates high risk)

Anti-arrhythmic	**Sotalol**
Anti-cancer	Tamoxifen
Anti-emetic	**Domperidone, ondansetron**, prochlorperazine, metoclopramide
Anti-fungal	**Fluconazole**, itraconazole, ketoconazole
Anti-hypertensive	Indapamide, bendroflumethiazide (by causing hypokalaemia)
Anti-migraine	Naratriptan, sumatriptan, zolmitriptan
Asthma inhalers	Salbutamol, salmeterol, terbutaline
Gastrointestinal	Esomeprazole, lansoprazole, omeprazole, loperamide
Macrolides	**Azithromycin, erythromycin, clarithromycin**
Mental health	**Amitriptyline, citalopram, chlorpromazine, escitalopram**, fluoxetine, **haloperidol**, hydroxyzine, lithium, quetiapine, paroxetine, risperidone, sertraline, trazodone, venlafaxine
Quinolones	**Ciprofloxacin, levofloxacin**, ofloxacin
Urological	Solifenacin, tolterodine
OTC	Nytol® (diphenhydramine), Sudafed® (pseudoephedrine), many cold remedies
Others	Metronidazole, quinine, furosemide

INTERACTIONS

A simple theoretical model, based purely on probability, shows that if the chance of an interaction between any two drugs is 1%, the chance of an interaction occurring when someone is taking 12 drugs is about 50%. Further prescribing will clearly increase this risk. Fortunately, many interactions are not serious; the prime aim is to avoid those that are. Warnings from clinical computer systems are helpful, but if you find your attention to such alerts wanes because of their frequency, consider changing the user settings to only alert you to a higher-priority problem.

Here are some examples of relevance to the management of minor illness (Table 14.3).

Table 14.3 Examples of long-term medications that interact with acute medications (bold type indicates high risk)

Long-term medication	Interacting acute medication for minor illness
Aspirin	NSAIDs – *increased risk of gastrointestinal haemorrhage and reduced cardiovascular protection*
Amiodarone	Colchicine – *increased toxicity*
Ciclosporin	Azithromycin, clarithromycin, fluconazole, itraconazole – *increased ciclosporin level* Colchicine – *increased toxicity* NSAIDs, trimethoprim – *increased renal toxicity*
Digoxin	Colchicine – *increased toxicity*
Lithium	NSAIDs – *increased lithium level*
Methotrexate	**Trimethoprim – *serious dual interference with folate metabolism*** NSAIDs – *increased methotrexate level*
Statin	Clarithromycin, fluconazole – *increased statin level and risk of rhabdomyolysis*
Theophylline	Clarithromycin, fluconazole, itraconazole, colchicine – *increased theophylline level*
Ticagrelor	Clarithromycin – *increased ticagrelor level*
Warfarin	NSAIDs – *enhanced anticoagulation and risk of gastrointestinal haemorrhage* Antibiotics (particularly clarithromycin), fluconazole, itraconazole, topical miconazole – *enhanced anticoagulation*

This table gives just a few examples of the many interactions that can occur, but take another look and see if you can spot a few themes (NSAIDs, colchicine, clarithromycin and fluconazole are a good starting point). Rather than trying to remember all the different interactions, it is more reliable to have a high index of suspicion for certain types of drug and check for possible interactions using the BNF (Box 14.2).

BOX 14.2 FACTORS THAT INCREASE THE RISK OF A SIGNIFICANT DRUG INTERACTION

- Drugs that share an effect – for example, aspirin and warfarin can both cause gastrointestinal bleeding
- Drugs that have opposite effects – for example, salbutamol will not be so effective if the patient is taking propranolol
- A drug that inhibits the metabolism of other drugs – for example, clarithromycin, fluconazole
- A drug that can affect renal function and the excretion of other drugs – for example, NSAIDs
- A drug that needs careful adjustment of dose or monitoring – for example, digoxin, methotrexate, lithium

---

Drugs that take a long time to be eliminated from the body (e.g. amiodarone, azithromycin, fluoxetine) can interact with other drugs several days or even weeks after they have been discontinued. You can suspect that a drug may have a long half-life if it is administered once a day or less often. This is not always the case, but it is useful as an alert; the actual half-life can then be checked in the SmPC (www.medicines.org.uk). Be wary of drugs that require careful dose adjustment (e.g. warfarin, ciclosporin, antiepileptics), as small effects from another drug on the metabolism can decrease the drug's effectiveness or increase its toxicity. A clue to recognising these drugs is that the blood levels are often monitored. Patients who are stabilised on very small doses may be at greater risk of a signficant interaction.

None of the antibiotics recommended in this book interact with oral contraceptives. In fact, the only antibiotics that do interact are the few that enhance the action of enzymes, such as some used to treat tuberculosis (Faculty of Sexual and Reproductive Healthcare Clinical Effectiveness Unit, 2017). There is no need to advise women taking antibiotics for minor illness to change their normal pill routine.

Not all interactions are from prescribed medication. St John's wort affects the metabolism of many other drugs, as does grapefruit juice. Cranberry juice increases the effect of warfarin, and alcohol interacts with metronidazole.

OTC

Drugs marked 'OTC' are available over the counter and often cost less than a prescription charge. The price depends on the pack size, brand and pharmacy; surprisingly the cost incurred by the NHS when prescribing such medicines can be far greater than purchase price for patients. In 2018, NHS England released guidance to Clinical Commissioning Groups aimed at reducing the prescribing of items available OTC, particularly for self-limiting conditions or those lending themselves to self-care. Even if the condition for which the medicine is required is not covered by this guidance, it is always worth enquiring whether the patient pays prescription charges and advising them accordingly.

BLACK TRIANGLE SYMBOL ▼

This symbol means that there is limited experience of the use of this product, and the Medicines and Healthcare Products Regulatory Agency (MHRA) requests that *all* suspected adverse reactions should be reported. Use the yellow forms in the BNF or at https://yellowcard.mhra.gov.uk/. They can be signed and submitted by any health professional, not just doctors.

FORMULATIONS

Clinical computer systems list available formulations of a drug. The main decision when prescribing for minor illness is to choose between a liquid and a solid tablet or capsule. It is often assumed that all children will need a liquid, but the work of the Canadian paediatrician Bonnie Kaplan showed that children as young as 4 years can be taught how to swallow solid forms easily (Kaplan et al., 2010). If a child is willing to try a solid form and has had experience of bad tasting liquids, consider offering a solid version of a medication.

Check the price of the formulation you are prescribing; you may be surprised. Nitrofurantoin liquid is £447 for 300 ml, according to the drug tariff at the time of publication, compared to £9.50 for a pack of nitrofurantoin MR tablets. Worse still may be medicines marked with no price at all or £0.00 (often a suspension or liquid formulation). These are likely to be 'specials' and can be incredibly expensive. It is not unheard of for thousands of pounds to be charged for a special that has been unwittingly prescribed, while a cheap alternative was easily available. Pharmacies often call to query such a prescription, but sadly, this is not always the case.

PACK SIZE

Aim to prescribe an amount that corresponds to a manufactured pack size. This may not necessarily be equal to the amount required for a full course. For example, a prescription for an antibiotic liquid can include an instruction to take it for a certain number of days, but the manufactured pack, which may contain more than is needed, can be dispensed whole, together with the patient information leaflet. Many of the items prescribed for minor illness are for short courses, but if a longer duration is needed, be aware that packs of tablets or capsules commonly contain 28 or 30. The regulations regarding packaging vary across regions.

DOSE

Where a medication is suggested in the text for management of a minor illness, the doses given will be appropriate for that illness. Other dosages and formulations may be available for other indications, a point worth bearing in mind when checking the medication in the BNF or other resource.

PRESCRIBING FOR CHILDREN

Children are not just small adults; their chemistry is still developing, and they may metabolise drugs quite differently. Some drugs that are safe for use by adults cannot be taken by children because of the risk of a side effect that only affects children – for example, aspirin may cause Reye's syndrome. For drugs that can be prescribed for children, the dose is usually calculated by weight. Calculating a dose by body surface area is more accurate, but using weight is much more practical (Box 14.3).

BOX 14.3 TIPS FOR SAFE PRESCRIBING FOR CHILDREN

- Use the BNFC
- Calculate the dose from the child's weight
- Be aware that if the child is heavy, this calculated dose might exceed the maximum dose recommended – adjust down – it should never be more than the adult dose
- Have an approximate idea of what the dose is likely to be – use this to check the calculation is correct or compare it with a dose for a given age range
- Note the instruction on how many doses per day
- If there appears to be no suitable formulation to make the dose easy to take (e.g. tiny or large amount of a liquid), recheck the calculation as there is likely to have been an error

---

It is helpful to have a rough idea of what you expect the dose to be before doing the calculation. If your result is very different from what you expect, then there is probably an error in the calculation. The rule of 4's helps to give an approximation: a dose for 14-year-old is similar to adult, and for every 4 years younger, the dose drops by one-fourth.

If no weighing scales are available, use the age-range dose in the BNFC or calculate according to the average weight-for-age table on the penultimate page of the book (or in the app under More > Guidance > Approximate Conversions and Units > Prescribing for children: weight, height, and gender). As a last resort, an approximate weight for a child aged 1–10 years can be calculated as (age + 4) × 2 kg, so a 6-year-old would weigh about 20 kg. This formula will give a weight to within 15% of the average weight of a child of that age.

Rounding up or down of a calculated dose may be necessary to make it practical. For example, the BNFC gives the dose of cefalexin for a child aged 5–11 years as '12.5 mg/kg twice daily, alternatively 250 mg three times a day'. Your 8-year-old patient weighs 25 kg, giving a calculated dose of 312.5 mg twice daily, which is more tailored to this particular child at their weight than the stated dose of 250 mg three times a day that covers all children in this age range. An oral suspension is available in a strength of 250 mg/5 mL, so your calculated dose would require 6.25 mL twice daily. Given the alternative in the BNFC, you can appreciate that the 0.25 mL represents an unnecessary degree of precision, so round the dose down to 6 mL twice daily. Obesity has an influence on this final adjustment of the dose. Most drugs do not penetrate fat well but are distributed within the water of the circulation and tissues. If a patient (of any age) is obese, calculating a dose by weight tends to give a dose that is rather too high, as the weight of the fat is included in the calculation, but most of the drug will be elsewhere. Conversely, a particularly thin patient may have a calculated dose that tends to err too low.

If you suspect an adverse drug reaction in anyone under the age of 18 years, it should be reported to the *MHRA* using the yellow form in the back of the BNF or at https://yellowcard.mhra.gov.uk/. This is because experience of use of the drug in children may still be limited.

PRESCRIBING IN PREGNANCY AND BREASTFEEDING

Every prescriber tries to avoid prescribing in pregnancy, but sometimes the risk from medication is outweighed by a greater risk of leaving a condition untreated, such as a urinary infection. Independent prescribers can prescribe for medical conditions presenting in pregnancy, so long as they work within their own level of professional competence (Royal College of Nursing, 2017). Before prescribing, always check the relevant section of text for the drug in the BNF that advises on risk in pregnancy or breastfeeding (Box 14.4).

BOX 14.4 FURTHER INFORMATION ON DRUG USE

In pregnancy:

UK Teratology Information Service (UKTIS) – www.uktis.org

In breastfeeding:

LactMed (USA) – toxnet.nlm.nih.gov/newtoxnet/lactmed.htm or download the free app

---

An observational study of 96,000 pregnant women in Canada (Muanda et al., 2017) found that women who were prescribed certain antibiotics in pregnancy had an increased rate of miscarriage. There was an increased risk for clarithromycin (odds ratio 2.35, number needed to harm 8) and azithromycin (odds ratio 1.65, number needed to harm 18). There was no increased risk for erythromycin. Subsequently, Public Health England (PHE) has recommended avoiding clarithromycin and azithromycin in pregnancy (PHE, 2017). When prescribing, remember that although erythromycin is the recommended macrolide for use in pregnancy, it still has the problems of multiple interactions, prolongation of the QT interval and delayed absorption when using the enteric-coated formulations. There is an alternative, which is often overlooked because of previous misinformation: cefalexin.

CEFALEXIN

The first cephalosporin was discovered in a sewage outflow in Sardinia in 1945. Perhaps this inauspicious beginning heralded the bad press these antibiotics later received. The two myths that have propagated through texts and the habits of prescribers are that all cephalosporins have a high risk of causing *Clostridium difficile*-associated diarrhoea (CDAD), and that because they have a beta-lactam ring like penicillins, they cannot be used if the patient is allergic to penicillin.

The first of these myths arose from a dumbing down of the correct realisation that later generations of cephalosporins, mostly used parenterally for inpatients, do indeed increase the risk of antibiotic-related enteritis. Cefalexin is a first-generation cephalosporin, but it was lumped together with all the rest in well-intentioned but inaccurate dissemination of the information gleaned from hospital care to primary care. The first alerts from the UK regulatory authorities specified a particular risk with third-generation cephalosporins, but this detail was lost in transit to prescribers. The only third-generation cephalosporin likely to be used in primary care in the United Kingdom is cefixime, and it is not recommended anywhere in this manual.

While many national campaigns were underway to dissuade prescribers from using any cephalosporin, Quentin Minson and Steve Mok (two American pharmacists) undertook a case-control study that examined the link between many different antibiotics and CDAD (Minson and Mok, 2007). They confirmed that third-generation cephalosporins carried a high risk (odds ratio 4.64), but that first-generation cephalosporins such as cefalexin turned out to have an odds ratio lower than 1 (it was 0.8 but the confidence interval included 1). Though the study was small and could be criticised for being underpowered, a subsequent meta-analysis found similar findings (Slimings and Riley, 2014). Indeed, current advice from NICE (2015) is that the risk seen with first generation cephalosporins, such as cefalexin, is not statistically significant, quoting the work of Slimings and Riley (2014) on subgroups of antibiotic classes that found an odds ratio for first-generation cephalosporins of 1.04 (confidence interval 0.88–1.24). Perversely, avoiding all cephalosporins meant that prescribers in primary care were having to choose an alternative antibiotic, and in doing so, they were often using broad-spectrum antibiotics actually known to be associated with CDAD, such as quinolones or co-amoxiclav.

The second misconception about cephalosporins resulted from a frequency of cross-sensitivity with penicillins of 10% quoted in earlier editions of the BNF, but the rate was falsely elevated by contamination of cephalosporins with penicillin during the manufacturing process used at the time. The presumption was that there would be a cross-sensitivity because both cephalosporins and penicillins share a beta-lactam ring in their molecular structure. There is cross-sensitivity, but now there is strong evidence that it results from not the ring but the R1 side-chain, which is similar in cefalexin, amoxicillin and ampicillin (Campagna et al., 2012). Estimates of the rate of cross-sensitivity vary (depending on the research method and type of cephalosporin studied) but a reasonable average is 4.3% (Lee, 2014). The rate of confirmed sensitivity to penicillin in those declaring themselves to have had a mild or moderate reaction to a penicillin is about 5.5% (Goldberg and Confino-Cohen, 2008). The chance of such a patient having a similar response to cefalexin is therefore 0.24%, or 1 in about 400. A very low rate has been found in clinical practice (Blumenthal et al., 2015; Goodman et al., 2001). People with a previous episode of immediate hypersensitivity (e.g. anaphylaxis) to penicillin or a cephalosporin should not receive either. Here the sensitivity is definite, and a cross-sensitivity rate of 4% is too high to risk another reaction.

PREVIOUS ANTIBIOTIC TREATMENT

If a patient presents with a condition requiring further antibiotic treatment but has received a course of the first-line antibiotic within the last 7 days, then either the infection is viral, or the organism is resistant to the antibiotic. If possible, take a sample for culture to discover which applies. If a different antibiotic is needed, then the second course needs to have a different or broader spectrum of antimicrobial activity. Reasonable switches are as follows, bearing in mind that you need to check that the substitute drug is suitable for the patient:

- For otitis media or sinusitis – change to co-amoxiclav
- For chest infections – add clarithromycin or change to doxycycline
- For uncomplicated urinary tract infections in non-pregnant women – if sensitivities are available from the laboratory, be guided by the results; otherwise use an antibiotic that was not used last time: nitrofurantoin MR, pivmecillinam, trimethoprim or fosfomycin
- For throat infections – take a throat swab and await the result before prescribing a different antibiotic as, in most cases, the infection will be viral

ROUTES OF DRUG ADMINISTRATION

Take advantage of the wide range of formulations of drugs. If a patient would benefit from a particular medication but there is potential risk or difficulty, consider using the drug via a different route of administration to the usual one, rather than changing to a less appropriate treatment. For example, a patient with a previous peptic ulcer presenting acutely with a soft tissue injury could use a topical NSAID rather than oral treatment. Be aware that an unusual formulation may be much more expensive than the usual one; note the example given earlier in this chapter of nitrofurantoin liquid (£447 for 300 mL). Paracetamol tablets are 2p each compared with £3.65 for a paracetamol suppository of the same dose. You can check the price of generic drugs online at www.ppa.org.uk/ppa/edt_intro.htm in Part VIII 'Basic Prices of Drug Product List'. The latest edition of *MIMS* gives an up-to-date price of branded products, but the BNF book price may be somewhat out-of-date because it is published less frequently. If you cannot find a form of a medicine in the BNF at all, it may be available but only supplied as a 'special' drug, without a set price, that could turn out to be thousands of pounds.

MEDICATION ADVICE

Dose of medication

The appropriate adult dose of medication for a condition is given in the text of this book. For the latest information, see the BNF and for children the BNFC.

Risk alerts for medications

Table 14.4 gives the abbreviations found after drug names in the text where there is a significant risk of adverse events. Any drug may have potential for multiple interactions, but the majority are not clinically significant. The tags provide warnings where there is a risk. Manufacturers often advise against the use of a medication in pregnancy or breastfeeding when there is insufficient evidence of safety. Independent information sources, such as the BNF, UK Teratology Information Service (UKTIS) and Drugs and Lactation Database (LactMed) may advise that there is no evidence of harm. A balance needs to be

Table 14.4 Prescribing symbols used in this book

P	**Pregnancy** risk. Use an alternative medication known to be safe in pregnancy. If the patient is allergic to penicillin, alternatives include cefalexin or erythromycin. Cefalexin, which shares some molecular structure with penicillins, should not be used if the patient has had an anaphylactic reaction to any penicillin. Erythromycin is preferred to clarithromycin or azithromycin if a macrolide is needed. Information sources: BNF or UKTIS.
B	**Breastfeeding** risk. The drug affects breastfeeding or is secreted in milk and is not suitable for the baby. Use an alternative medication known to be safe in breastfeeding. Information sources: BNF or LactMed.
C	**Children.** The medication is either harmful to children or has a limited licence, for example, the medicine may only be licensed for children over a certain age. Information source: BNFC.
I	**Interactions** likely. For example, macrolides such as clarithromycin inhibit the liver enzymes that metabolise drugs. This can result in an accumulation of another drug to potentially toxic levels. Many drugs can be affected (e.g. amlodipine, colchicine, simvastatin, ticagrelor, warfarin), so always check the BNF for any interaction before prescribing. If a macrolide is needed, but clarithromycin is precluded because of interactions, consider azithromycin, which does not interact significantly with the hepatic cytochrome P450 system. Information sources: BNF or EMC.
Q	**QT interval** prolonged. Avoid for anyone with a known long QT interval, an unknown QT interval plus a family history of unexplained sudden death, or for anyone already taking another drug that prolongs the interval. A long interval between the Q and T waves on an ECG indicate an increased risk of cardiac arrhythmias that can cause sudden death. Information sources: SADS or CredibleMeds.

Websites
BNF: bnf.nice.org.uk
BNFC: bnfc.nice.org.uk
CredibleMeds: www.crediblemeds.org
EMC: www.medicines.org.uk
LactMed: toxnet.nlm.nih.gov/newtoxnet/lactmed.htm
SADS: www.sads.org.uk
UKTIS: www.uktis.org

struck to avoid denying pregnant or lactating women helpful medication whilst maintaining adequate safety for the foetus or infant.

The tags to each drug name may vary depending on the context. For example, oral prednisolone is suitable for use in asthma for a pregnant woman where the benefit outweighs the risk, but not when it is being considered as an option to treat hay fever.

It should be remembered that the elimination of many drugs can be affected by renal or hepatic impairment. If the patient has either, check the dose of the drug in the relevant section of the BNF/BNFC.

These symbols are designed to alert you quickly and simply to prescribing issues which are common and important. They cannot cover all possibilities; full information on prescribing is available in the BNF and BNFC.

References

Avery, T., Barber, N., Ghaleb, M., Franklin, B.D., Armstrong, S., Crowe, S., Dhillon, S., et al. 2012. Investigating the prevalence and causes of prescribing errors in general practice: The PRACtICe Study. (PRevalence and Causes of prescrIbing errors in general practiCe). *A report for the GMC.* www.gmc-uk.org/about/what-we-do-and-why/data-and-research/research-and-insight-archive/investigating-the-prevalence-and-causes-of-prescribing-errors-in-general-practice.

Blumenthal, K.G., Shenoy, E.S., Varughese, C.A., Hurwitz, S., Hooper, D.C., and Banerji, A. 2015. Impact of a clinical guideline for prescribing antibiotics to inpatients reporting penicillin or cephalosporin allergy. *Ann Allergy Asthma Immunol* 2015; 115(4):294–300.e2. www.annallergy.org/article/S1081-1206(15)00336-1/fulltext. doi: 10.1016/j.anai.2015.05.011.

Boggiano, B.G., and Gleeson, M. 1976. Gastric acid inactivation of erythromycin stearate in solid dosage forms. *J Pharm Sci*; 65(4):497–502. jpharmsci.org/article/S0022-3549(15)40712-9/pdf.

Campagna, J.D., Bond, M.C., Schabelman, E., and Hayes, B.D. 2012. The use of cephalosporins in penicillin-allergic patients: A literature review. *The Journal of Emergency Medicine*; 42(5):612–620. www.jem-journal.com/article/S0736-4679(11)00545-2/fulltext.

Faculty of Sexual and Reproductive Healthcare Clinical Effectiveness Unit. 2017. *Drug interactions with hormonal contraception.* www.fsrh.org/pdfs/CEUGuidanceDrugInteractionsHormonal.pdf.

Goldberg, A., and Confino-Cohen, R. 2008. Skin testing and oral penicillin challenge in patients with a history of remote penicillin allergy. *Annals of Allergy, Asthma & Immunology*; 100(1):37–43. www.sciencedirect.com/science/article/pii/S1081120610604024.

Goodman, E.J., Morgan, M.J., Johnson, P.A., Nichols, B.A., Denk, N., and Gold, B.B. 2001. Cephalosporins can be given to penicillin-allergic patients who do not exhibit an anaphylactic response. *Journal of Clinical Anesthesia*; 13(8): 561–564. www.jcafulltextonline.com/article/S0952-8180(01)00329-4/fulltext.

Kaplan, B.J. 2010. *The new method of swallowing.* www.youtube.com/watch?v=MXFMZuNs-Fk; www.research4kids/pillswallowing.

Kaplan, B.J., Steiger, R.A., Pope, J., Marsh, A., Sharp, M., and Crawford, S.G. 2010. Successful treatment of pill-swallowing difficulties with head posture practice. *Paediatr Child Health (online)*; 15: 1–5. academic.oup.com/pch/article/15/5/e1/2639510/ Successful-treatment-of-pill-swallowing.

Lee, Q.U. 2014. Use of cephalosporins in patients with immediate penicillin hypersensitivity: cross-reactivity revisited. *Hong Kong Med J*; 20(5):428–436. www.hkmj.org/abstracts/v20n5/428.htm. doi: 10.12809/hkmj144327.

Minson, Q., and Mok, S. 2007. Relationship between antibiotic exposure and subsequent Clostridium difficile-associated diarrhoea. *Hosp Pharm*; 42(5):430–434.

Muanda, F.T., Sheehy, O., and Bérard, A. 2017. Use of antibiotics during pregnancy and risk of spontaneous abortion. *Canadian Medical Association Journal*; 189(17):E625–E633. www.ncbi.nlm.nih.gov/pmc/articles/PMC5415390/.

NHS England. 2018. Conditions for which over the counter items should not routinely be prescribed in primary care: Guidance for CCGs. www.england.nhs.uk/publication/conditions-for-which-over-the-counter-items-should-not-routinely-be-prescribed-in-primary-care-guidance-for-ccgs/

NICE. 2015. Clostridium difficile infection: Risk with broad-spectrum antibiotics. www.nice.org.uk/advice/esmpb1/chapter/Key-points-from-the-evidence.

Oscanoa, T.J., Lizaraso, F., and Carvajal, A. 2017. Hospital admissions due to adverse drug reactions in the elderly. A meta-analysis. *European Journal of Clinical Pharmacology*; 73(6): 759–770. https://link.springer.com/article/10.1007%2Fs00228-017-2225-3.

Public Health England. 2017. Management and treatment of common infections. www.gov.uk/government/publications/managing-common-infections-guidance-for-primary-care

Royal College of Nursing. 2017. *Prescribing in pregnancy.* www.rcn.org.uk/clinical-topics/medicines-optimisation/specialist-areas/prescribing-in-pregnancy.

Slimings, C., and Riley, T.V. 2014. Antibiotics and hospital-acquired Clostridium difficile infection: Update of systematic review and meta-analysis. *Journal of Antimicrobial Chemotherapy*; 69(4): 881–891. https://academic.oup.com/jac/article/69/4/881/705659/Antibiotics-and-hospital-acquired-Clostridium.

Tamma, P.D., Avdic, E., Li, D.L., Dzintars, K., and Cosgrove, S.E. 2017. Association of adverse events with antibiotic use in hospitalized patients. *JAMA Intern Med*;177(9): 1308–1315.

CHAPTER 15

Resources

REFERENCE BOOKS

British National Formulary (BNF) – updated every 6 months and published by the British Medical Association (BMA) and Royal Pharmaceutical Society of Great Britain. Make sure you are not using an out-of-date copy! Instead give it to Pharmaid commonwealthpharmacy.org Tel: +44 (0) 7761 574284 email: admin@commonwealthpharmacy.org. The BNF and BNFC are available online at bnf.nice.org.uk. You can download the BNF and BNFC apps to your phone without cost or password from the App Store or Play Store.

OTC Directory – published annually by the Proprietary Society of Great Britain. Details (and pictures) of many common over-the-counter preparations. Obtain the book from www.pagb.co.uk/self-care/otcdirectory.

OTHER READING

Ashton, R., Leppard, B., and Cooper, H. 2014. *Differential Diagnosis in Dermatology*, 4th edition. CRC Press. ISBN-13:978-1909368729.
   This book has very useful algorithms that explain the likely diagnoses for a particular presentation and their distinguishing features.
Beckwith, S., and Franklin, P. 2011. *Oxford Handbook of Prescribing for Nurses and Allied Health Professionals*, 2nd edition. Oxford University Press. ISBN-13: 978-0199575817.
Guillebaud, J. 2017. *Contraception, Your Questions Answered*, 7th edition. Elsevier. ISBN-13: 978-0702070006.
Neal, M.J. 2015. *Medical Pharmacology at a Glance*, 8th edition. Wiley-Blackwell. ISBN-13: 978-1118902400.
Nuttall, D., and Rutt-Howard, J. 2015. *The Textbook of Non-Medical Prescribing*. Wiley-Blackwell. ISBN-13: 78-1118856499.
Rushforth, H. 2012. *Assessment Made Incredibly Easy*, 5th edition. Lippincott, Williams & Wilkins. ISBN-13: 978-1451147278.

ONLINE

www.minorillness.co.uk: *Our own NMIC website.*

There should be a voucher in the front of this book that will give you 6 months' free access to the members' section, with online educational materials and email alerts.

Scan this QR code with your smartphone to take you there directly.

cks.nice.org.uk: *The most useful site for detailed, evidence-based advice on minor illness*

patient.info: *A good source of patient information leaflets and self-help groups*

www.evidence.nhs.uk: *Many useful resources, including the BNF and the Cochrane Library*

www.tripdatabase.com: *For the answer to that awkward question*

labtestsonline.org: *For advice about laboratory tests*

www.pcds.org.uk: *Diagnostic algorithms for skin conditions*

www.dermnetnz.org: *For images and management of skin conditions* www.rcgp.org.uk/clinical-and-research/resources/toolkits/target-antibiotic-toolkit.aspx: *Downloadable Target Toolkit forms for patients*

www.publichealth.hscni.net/publications/guidance-infection-control-schools-and-other-childcare-settings-0:   *For information on infectiousness and school exclusion. This poster is for Northern Ireland – unfortunately the UK version is currently unavailable*

www.gov.uk/government/collections/immunisation-against-infectious-disease-the-green-book: *Current immunisation schedules and the 'Green Book: Immunisation against Infectious Disease'*

www.spottingthesickchild.com: *Detailed advice on the assessment of children*

www.whenshouldiworry.com: *An evidence-based booklet for parents on respiratory infections*

www.nice.org.uk: *National guidance on a wide range of conditions*

nathnac.net: *Travel advice*

www.travax.scot.nhs.uk: *Up-to-date advice about travel vaccination and malaria*

www.dwp.gov.uk/fitnote: *Information about MED3 certificates*

www.bashh.org: *Information and guidelines on sexual health*

europepmc.org: *For free access to millions of publications*

www.arthritisresearchuk.org: *Exercise sheets for common musculoskeletal pains*

PRESCRIBING INFORMATION SOURCES

Internet resources

Source	Website
British National Formulary	bnf.nice.org.uk *App also available*
OTC Drug Information	otcdirectory.pagb.co.uk
Electronic Medicines Compendium	www.medicines.org.uk *Patient information leaflet (PIL) and Summary of Product Characteristics (SmPC) including frequencies of side effects and half-life*
Monthly Index of Medical Specialities	www.mims.co.uk *Pharmaceutically sponsored, but is up-to-date, more succinct than the BNF and has useful tables, for example, emollient additives*
The Cochrane Library	www.cochranelibrary.com
PubMed medical database	europepmc.org
Specialist Pharmacy Service	www.sps.nhs.uk *Professional medicines advice*
UKTIS	www.uktis.org *Prescribing information in pregnancy*
LactMed	toxnet.nlm.nih.gov/newtoxnet/lactmed.htm *Prescribing information for breastfeeding mothers. App also available*
SADS	www.sads.org.uk *UK information on QT interval*
CredibleMeds	www.crediblemeds.org *US information on QT interval*
University of Indiana	medicine.iupui.edu/clinpharm/ddis/ *Information on cytochrome P450 drug interactions*

Many of the best and most up-to-date information sources are on the Internet, either freely available or available with an NHS Athens password via www.evidence.nhs.uk.

CHAPTER 16

Abbreviations

5-HT	5-hydroxytryptamine
A&E	Accident and Emergency Department
ACE	angiotensin-converting enzyme
ADR	adverse drug reaction
AI	artificial intelligence
ARB	angiotensin receptor blocker
BMI	body mass index
BNF	British National Formulary
BNFC	British National Formulary for Children
BP	blood pressure
BTS	British Thoracic Society
BV	bacterial vaginosis
CBT	cognitive behavioural therapy
CCB	calcium channel blocker
CCG	Clinical Commissioning Group
CD	controlled drug
CDAD	*Clostridium difficile*-associated diarrhoea
C. difficile	*Clostridium difficile*
CKD	chronic kidney disease
CKS	Clinical Knowledge Summaries
CNS	central nervous system
COC	combined oral contraceptive
COPD	chronic obstructive pulmonary disease
CRB-65	a scoring system for pneumonia
CRP	C-reactive protein, an inflammatory marker in the blood
CRT	capillary refill time
CXR	chest x-ray
DMARD	disease-modifying anti-rheumatic drug
doi	digital object identifier (a stable link to websites)
DVLA	Driver and Vehicle Licensing Agency
EC	emergency contraception
ECG	electrocardiogram
eGFR	estimated glomerular filtration rate
EMC	Electronic Medicines Compendium
ENT	Ear, Nose and Throat
ESR	erythrocyte sedimentation rate
FBC	full blood count
FPG	fasting plasma glucose
FSRH	Faculty of Sexual and Reproductive Healthcare
G6PD	glucose-6-phosphate dehydrogenase
GABHS	group A beta-haemolytic *Streptococcus*
GCS	Glasgow coma scale
GDP	gross domestic product
GI	gastrointestinal
GP	General Practitioner
HADS	Hospital Anxiety and Depression Scale
HbA1c	Haemoglobin A1c, a marker for level of glycaemia over the past 3 months

HFMD	hand, foot and mouth disease
HIV	human immunodeficiency virus
HPT	health protection team
H. pylori	*Helicobacter pylori*
HRT	hormone replacement therapy
HSP	Henoch-Schönlein purpura
HVS	high vaginal swab
IBD	inflammatory bowel disease
ICS	Integrated Care System
IM	intramuscular
IT	information technology
IUCD	intrauterine contraceptive device
IUS	intrauterine system
IV	intravenous
LFT	liver function tests
LMP	last menstrual period
MAOI	monoamine oxidase inhibitor
MDI	metered-dose inhaler
MED3	certificate of fitness for work
Men B	meningitis B
MHRA	Medicines and Healthcare Products Regulatory Agency
MIMS	Monthly Index of Medical Specialties
MMR	measles, mumps and rubella
MR	modified-release
MRSA	methicillin-resistant *Staphylococcus aureus*
MSU	midstream urine
NAAT	nucleic acid amplification test
NHS	National Health Service
NICE	National Institute for Health and Care Excellence
NMC	Nursing & Midwifery Council
NMIC	National Minor Illness Centre
NNT	number needed to treat
NSAID	non-steroidal anti-inflammatory drug
ORS	oral rehydration solution
OTC	over-the-counter
PCDS	Primary Care Dermatology Society
PEFR	peak expiratory flow rate
pH	a measure of acidity
PHQ-9	Patient Health Questionnaire 9
PHE	Public Health England
POP	progestogen-only pill
PoTS	postural tachycardia syndrome
PPI	proton pump inhibitor
QT	part of an ECG trace
RA	rheumatoid arthritis
RCGP	Royal College of General Practitioners
RCOG	Royal College of Obstetricians and Gynaecologists
RR	respiratory rate
SADS	sudden arrhythmic death syndrome
SGLT2	sodium-glucose linked transporter type 2
SIGN	Scottish Intercollegiate Guidelines Network
SmPC	Summary of Product Characteristics (of a medicine)
SSRI	selective serotonin reuptake inhibitor
STI	sexually transmitted infection
STP	Sustainability and Transformation Partnership
TB	tuberculosis
TENS	transcutaneous electrical nerve stimulation

ToP	termination of pregnancy
TTG	tissue transglutaminase (a blood test for coeliac disease)
TV	*Trichomonas vaginalis*
UK	United Kingdom
UKTIS	UK Teratology Information Service
UPSI	unprotected sexual intercourse
URTI	upper respiratory tract infection
UTI	urinary tract infection
VTE	venous thromboembolism
VZIG	*varicella zoster* immunoglobulin
WHO	World Health Organisation

Index